PSYCHIATRIC
DIAGNOSIS

Psychiatric Diagnosis

Edited by

Vivian M. Rakoff, M.A., M.B.B.S., F.R.C.P.(C)

Professor of Psychiatric Education
Department of Psychiatry
University of Toronto

Harvey C. Stancer, Ph.D., M.D., F.R.C.P.(C)

Professor of Psychiatric Research
Department of Psychiatry
University of Toronto

and

Henry B. Kedward, M.A., M.D., F.R.C.P.(C)

Professor, Department of Psychiatry
University of Toronto

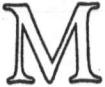

© Brunner/Mazel, Inc., 1977
Softcover reprint of the hardcover 1st edition 1977

All rights reserved. No part of this publication
may be reproduced or transmitted, in any form or
by any means, without permission

First published in the United States of America 1977
by Brunner/Mazel, Inc., New York

Published in Great Britain 1978 by
THE MACMILLAN PRESS LTD
London and Basingstoke
Associated companies in Delhi Dublin
Hong Kong Johannesburg Lagos Melbourne
New York Singapore and Tokyo

British Library Cataloguing in Publication Data

Psychiatric diagnosis.
　1. Mental illness - Diagnosis
　I. Rakoff, Vivian M　II. Stancer, Harvey C
　III. Kedward, Henry B
　616.89′075　　　　RC469

ISBN 978-1-349-03755-1　　　ISBN 978-1-349-03753-7 (eBook)
DOI 10.1007/978-1-349-03753-7

Contents

Contributors

JEAN ENDICOTT, Ph.D.

Assistant Professor of Clinical Psychology, Department of Psychiatry, College of Physicians and Surgeons, Columbia University; Member, Task Force on Nomenclature and Statistics of the American Psychiatric Association

ALVAN R. FEINSTEIN, M.D.

Professor of Medicine and Epidemiology, Yale University School of Medicine

ROY R. GRINKER, SR., M.D.

Chairman of the Department of Psychiatry of Michael Reese Hospital

H. M. VAN PRAAG, M.D.

Professor of Psychiatry, Biological Psychiatry, State University, Groningen, Holland

RALPH M. REITAN, Ph.D.

Professor of Psychology and Neurological Surgery, University of Washington

MICHAEL SHEEHY, M.D.

Director of Outpatient Services and Research, Columbia Presbyterian-New York State Psychiatric Institute; Member, Task Force on Nomenclature and Statistics of the American Psychiatric Association

ROBERT L. SPITZER, M.D.

Professor of Clinical Psychiatry, Columbia University; Chairman, Task Force on Nomenclature and Statistics of the American Psychiatric Association

ROBERT J. STOLLER, M.D.

Professor, Department of Psychiatry, University of California School of Medicine, Los Angeles

PAUL H. WENDER, M.D.

Professor of Psychiatry, University of Utah, College of Medicine, Salt Lake City, Utah

JOHN K. WING, M.D., Ph.D.

Professor of Social Psychiatry, The Institute of Psychiatry, University of London, England

GEORGE WINOKUR, M.D.

Professor and Head, Department of Psychiatry, University of Iowa College of Medicine

Introduction

In common with the terms used in medicine and surgery, psychiatric diagnostic labels are derived from a ragbag of conceptual models: Diagnoses may be the names of symptoms, syndromes, signs or biochemical entities or historical relics—a received shorthand for complex states. But psychiatry has suffered more than its companion healing arts from a lack of generally accepted theoretical approaches or even commonly accepted empirical practice which could have provided the basis of a professional lingua franca. And even widely used terms may be applied very differently in different places, as the well-known U.S./U.K. study demonstrated. In some instances the problem is something like the situation encountered with languages such as Arabic, in which there is a language of usage so different from the formal language of literature that the ordinary man-in-the-street can barely follow the meaning of the literary language. In psychiatry this takes the form of the gap between elaborate diagnostic codes used for research purposes by epidemiologists and others and the limited repertoire of diagnoses used by the work-a-day clinician which rarely go beyond schizophrenia, depression, anxiety state, addiction, organic state, personality disorder, or neurosis.

At any particular moment in history diagnostic labeling can only be as good as the prevailing technology or, failing that, the prevailing accepted philosophy. Yet, allowing for all the uncertainty and confusion, psychiatric diagnosis in general is not as good as it could be, in the sense that it has not, at this time, incorporated recent advances in the associated sciences and disciplines—so that usage trails behind available knowledge.

There is in psychiatry very little well-based knowledge of pathogenesis; this is a situation that is fairly common in the history of the healing professions. However, in medicine and surgery there have frequently been effective therapies for maladies that have been poorly understood in terms of their causes and pathology. There is little of this pragmatic comfort for the psychiatrist since part of the problem is also the paucity of objectively defined therapeutic modalities of predictable effectiveness. The great majority of patients who traditionally present their suffering to psychiatrists fall into the framework of life problems or the loosely defined neuroses. The therapies for such conditions are usually psychotherapies of one kind or the other. For more severe psychiatric conditions, therapeutic practice begins with (or is based upon) prescription of phenothiazines, anti-depressants, anxiolytics, and lithium. The small range of materia medica more accurately reflects the pragmatic diagnostic labels referred to above rather than the elaborate grids and cross references encountered in classifications, such as the schedules of the World Health Organisation's diagnostic codes or the carefully researched versions of the Diagnostic and Statistical Manual (DSM) of the American Psychiatric Association.

The organisers of the symposium from which this book is derived planned to deal with the issue of psychiatric diagnosis from a range of points of view informing current practice. The intention was to examine each approach in terms of its advantages and shortcomings. We were particularly concerned to avoid diagnostic schemata based upon purely theoretical or speculative positions unsupported by empirical evidence. However, we were aware, as Dr. Wing writes, that all diagnostic categories, no matter how utilitarian or empirically derived, contain hypotheses which may or may not be explicit, or which may or may not have been subject to investigation.

We also attempted to structure the symposium to reflect not only conceptual variety but in a crude sense a hierarchy of diagnostic concerns and possibilities. We planned to have contributions ranging from the most palpably objective techniques of diagnosis through the application of the basic clinical and epidemiological sciences to the consideration of the patient's subjective motivational states. And having done that, we hoped to consider the "summa" of present knowledge as it is reflected in diagnostic schedules covering the entire range of adult psychiatric disorder.

The reader will find two descriptions of complete psychiatric diagnostic schedules: Dr. Spitzer and his colleagues have presented the problems involved in constructing DSM-III which will become the new standard nomenclature for North American psychiatrists. As Dr. Spitzer explains, it is essentially an attempt to rationalise North American usage. It adopts a multiaxial approach flexible enough to allow for multiple diagnoses arranged in a hierarchy of importance at any particular moment that the patient happens to present. It attempts to be as operational as possible in its naming and classification of disorders, and it may surprise the ordinary practitioner by its rejection of such hallowed daily terms as "the neuroses." As Dr. Spitzer writes, the version of the DSM-III published in broad outline in this text is still only in the nature of a working document which still has to be threshed through the dialectical process of detailed acceptance and rejection by various committees and pressure groups within the American psychiatric context.

Dr. John Wing, who has devoted many years to the standardisation of the psychiatric diagnostic process, describes the development and use of the standardised *Present State Examination* and the development of diagnostic criteria for international use. Dr. Wing is careful to remind the reader that even well researched systems of classification, which attempt to be as complete as possible, may not do justice to many of the difficulties patients will insist upon bringing to their physicians. In the panel discussion at the end of the conference he notes that political pressures may also affect the construction of diagnostic categories. As Dr. Spitzer has had to be responsive to the demands of American psychiatrists, so Dr. Wing and the international committees of the World Health Organisation have to be responsive to the variations in usage in several countries.

North American psychiatry has grown to maturity during a period in which the theoretical structures of psychoanalysis have been widely accepted. Dr. Robert Stoller has examined those concepts which he believes are relevant in considering psychiatric diagnostic categories. His particular concern is to put to one side some of the psychoanalytic theoretical constructs which may be difficult to apply to formal diagnosis. However, he emphasises that diagnoses based entirely upon behavioural or chemical phenomenology may ignore the varieties of motivation that may underlie similar clinical expression. The differences in motivation he proposes are essential for differentiating between diagnostc categories. These distinctions are not purely theoretical but have implications for treatment and prognosis. He chooses as his specific example the great variety of motivation in the matter of transvestism and transsexuality.

Psychiatry hopes for economical and precise clinical tests that will remove diagnosis from its present plane of uncertainty. Dr. Reitan in his chapter considers the use that may be made of neuropsychological concepts. He shows how the original work of Halstead has been applied so as to derive useful information through the vehicle of sophisticated psychological tests. Unfortunately, the range of diagnoses to which those techniques may be applied is still limited, but the precision and care that Dr. Reitan brings to the task remains an inspiration for most of our concerns.

It would be foolish to believe that much of our concern is not involved in polemic. Not only is there the polemical interchange of different points of view within the profession, but outside psychiatry there are critics who call into question the entire process of diagnosis and labeling. Dr. Roy Grinker, Sr. is concerned with keeping psychiatry within the framework of an effective and practical healing occupation. He opposes those who attempt to reject useful, albeit imperfect, diagnostic categories, and he gives an account of the work he and his associates have done in the notoriously difficult field of the borderline syndromes. (As readers will observe, the panel discussion spent a disproportionate amount of time in considering the problems raised by any diagnosis in which the word "borderline" appears.) Dr. Grinker, in his paper, outlines the process of matching clinical evidence, separating into coherent groups and arriving at an operational definition, which may be given to as problematic a category as the borderline syndrome. He insists that this label is valid and that it represents an example of the application of clinical experience and empirical method to a field that could easily be (and perhaps is) a morass. Dr. Feinstein wonders, in the panel discussion, whether the term borderline is appropriate at any time, comparing it with an analogous term such as borderline pregnancy. However, one feels inclined to remind the reader of the problems of internal medicine where incipient or subclinical syndromes such as diabetes seem analogous to some of the concepts of borderline as applied to psychiatric syndromes.

Both Drs. Wender and Winokur use genetic studies to cast light on subvarieties within a particular group of clinical disorders. Dr. Wender approaches the problem of schizophrenia and its apparently associated disorders which may represent formes frustes of the condition. He describes genetic studies and the clinical examination of families of schizophrenic probands, to cast light on the notion of the schizophrenia spectrum concept. Similarly Dr. Winokur describes how careful genetic studies of his well-known Iowa 500 have helped him and his colleagues to differentiate subvarieties within the affective disorders. At the same time he describes their search for "markers" that may be found in the laboratory which, while they may not be components of the disorders, may be signposts to them. His conclusions and techinques are subjected to critical examination in the panel discussion.

Dr. Herman van Praag suggests a different strategy for the use of laboratory data. And as Dr. Reitan was able to describe a limited series of neuropsychological tests to illuminate certain conditions, Dr. van Praag puts forward the idea that the measurement of metabolites of the biogenic amines in body fluids, such as the CSF, may be "markers" and help to differentiate the affective disorders so as to make pharmacotherapy more specific—and hence more efficient. It is one of the few areas within psychiatry where basic biological science has been utilised for clinical gain. Even in this area Dr. van Praag is aware that problems of terminological usage still remain a dilemma and that the differences in nosological practices in Europe and America still require constant research.

As Dr. Grinker criticised psychiatric usage from the point of view of a practitioner and researcher within the field, Dr. Alvan Feinstein brings to psychiatry the critical attention of someone who is more generally concerned with matters of medical diagnosis. It will gratify the practising mental health professional and perhaps surprise other critics to find that Dr. Feinstein sees very real analogies and similarities between the diagnostic problems faced by general physicians and those found in psychiatry. He places a constant search for scientifically derived categories within the continuing historical push towards objective fact and he reminds us that one cannot exist in advance of one's particular moment in history.

Considering the symposium as a whole, it appears as if we are on the verge of breakthroughs in the biological and genetic sphere, bringing us closer to defining some aspects of psychiatry as disease entities. What has been formerly labeled functional disorder may soon be constricted, or disappear, to be replaced by syndromes with a known pathophysiology and specific therapies. Yet it is equally apparent that we cannot forget the multitude of psychodynamic components which comprise what we call the personality. Much of the new information is already finding its way into the new diagnostic formulations of DSM-III and through good international liaison we can look forward to a similar incorporation into the I.C.D. Perhaps most important is the realisation that the investigation of psychiatric diagnoses is constantly in process. And this restless activity makes one hopeful for the future of psychiatry within medicine and science.

PSYCHIATRIC
DIAGNOSIS

1

DSM-III: Guiding Principles

ROBERT L. SPITZER, M.D., MICHAEL SHEEHY, M.D., and JEAN ENDICOTT, PH.D.

In September, 1973 a new Task Force on Nomenclature and Statistics of the American Psychiatric Association was constituted to develop the Third Edition of the American Psychiatric Association's *Diagnostic and Statistical Manual* (DSM-III). This conference is an opportune time to discuss the principles that have guided the Task Force. Many of these principles are clear to us now only as we step back and review the logic implicit in the countless decisions that we have made. As these principles become more explicit, they can guide subsequent work and provide standards for review of what already has been accomplished.

The Task Force's goal has been to develop a classification system that would reflect our current state of knowledge regarding mental disorders, and only secondarily to insure its compatibility with the chapter on Mental Disorders of the *International Classification of Diseases*. The original timetable scheduled publication of DSM-III in January, 1979 to coincide with introduction throughout this country of a clinical modification of the Ninth Edition of the *International Classification of Diseases* (ICD-9-CM). More recently, there has been a discussion as to the wisdom of extending field trials of DSM-II beyond that time in order to refine the system on the basis of extensive clinical use prior to its official adoption by the American Psychiatric Association.

1

This work is not the product of a small isolated committee. Although the Task Force itself now numbers 12 individuals, work on DSM-III has involved 10 advisory committees for portions of the nomenclature* and well over 100 individuals with special expertise in different areas of psychiatric diagnosis. Although many contributors are primarily academic or research psychiatrists or psychologists, there is ample representation of psychiatrists with predominantly clinical activities. As the work has progressed, it has been presented at several local and national professional meetings. A special conference was held in St. Louis, Missouri in June of 1976 to examine DSM-III in midstream. This conference, co-sponsored by the American Psychiatric Association and the Missouri Institute of Psychiatry, was attended by approximately 100 individuals who had expertise or special interest in various aspects of the classification. Several national mental health associations sent representatives, as well. Sessions at this conference were devoted to discussion of work to date on the major subdivisions of the classification. As a result of these discussions, additional diagnostic categories were added, some were deleted, and a decision was made to proceed with the development of multiaxial diagnosis. A number of new individuals became actively involved in the work of the Task Force, extending its efforts to areas such as Adolescent and Reactive Disorders. Formal liaison committees are now being set up with a large number of professional organizations representing psychiatry, psychoanalysis, medicine, neurology, pediatrics, psychology and social work, all of which have an interest in the development of DSM-III.

Multipurpose Classification

From the outset, the Task Force has assumed that in medicine an effective classification has many purposes. It is first a means by which the profession communicates briefly and clearly within itself about clinically recognizable conditions for which it has professional responsibility for diagnosis, care or research. Secondly, when possible, the classification should be a useful guide to current differentiated treatments. A third purpose is to provide information about the likely outcome of the psychiatric disorders with and without treatment. Finally, the classification should reflect what is known about the etiology or pathophysiological

---

* Organic Brain Disorders, Drug Use Disorders, Schizophrenia and Affective Disorders, Anxiety Disorders, Somatoform Disorders, Personality Disorders, Sexual Disorders, Psychosomatic Disorders, Child and Adolescent Disorders, Reactive Disorders.

processes involved in the disorders. When the etiology of a disorder is not known, as is the case with most of the mental disorders, the classification should facilitate systematic inquiry.

A Classification for the Entire Profession

Every effort is being made to develop DSM-III so that it will meet the needs of the entire psychiatric profession. This includes office practitioners, clinicians in institutional settings, research investigators, educators, and administrators. Each of these groups has special needs which at times may conflict. For example, the clinician frequently wishes to include categories in the diagnostic system which represent a consensus of clinical judgment and experience. On the other hand, research investigators are often reluctant to include diagnostic categories that have not been validated as distinct conditions by carefully controlled studies involving such variables as familial incidence, outcome (1), and treatment response (4). Administrators are most concerned with the implications of diagnostic terms in the areas of third party payments, forensic psychiatry, and legislative action.

Inclusiveness

Because the DSM-III classification is intended for the entire profession, and because our current knowledge about mental disorder is so limited, the Task Force has chosen to be inclusive rather than exclusive. In practice, this means that whenever a clinical condition can be described with clarity and relative distinctness, it is considered for inclusion. If there is general agreement among clinicians, who would be expected to encounter the condition, that there are a significant number of patients who have it and that its identification is important in their clinical work, it is included in the classification.

Mental Disorder Not Synonymous with Bad or Deviant Behavior

Efforts on the part of some members of the Task Force to arrive at a comprehensive definition of mental disorder have been deemed generally less than satisfactory (6). However, these efforts have made explicit some of the principles that have been applied in determining which conditions are included in DSM-III as mental disorders, and which are variants of human behavior outside the direct professional responsibility of the psychiatric profession. These principles help to avoid an overly broad definition of mental disorders that would view all individual and social unrest or problems of living as psychiatric illness, and at the same time justify the designation of mental disorders as a subset of medical disorders.

By and large, all of the conditions included in DSM-III as mental disorders share the following features: in their extreme or fully developed form, they are directly associated with either distress, disability, or, in the absence of either of these, disadvantage in coping with unavoidable aspects of the environment. Furthermore, they are not quickly ameliorated by simple nontechnical environmental maneuvers or informative procedures and do not have widespread social support. Because of these features, there is an implicit assumption that something is wrong with the human organism and there is a call to the profession to develop and offer preventive or therapeutic measures. (This does not imply exclusive responsibility on the part of the psychiatric profession to deal with these conditions.)

Three examples of the application of these principles in defining mental disorder follow. Personality disorders are included in DSM-III as mental disorders and are distinguished from personality traits (which are not included) on the basis of the presence of either subjective distress or impairment in social functioning. Simple bereavement is not considered a mental disorder, even though the clinical features are very similar to those seen in depressive disorders, because it is an expected and socially supported reaction. Finally, antisocial behavior is not by itself considered sufficient evidence for the existence of a mental disorder. The diagnosis of *Antisocial Personality Disorder* in DSM-III not only requires persistent antisocial behavior but also persistent impairment in social and occupational functioning.

Levels of Comprehension

Categorization in medicine can be usefully divided into three levels of comprehension. At the simplest level, an isolated sign or symptom is noted without any reference to the context in which it occurs. Examples are cough or depressed mood, which occur in many conditions. At the second level, there is a distinctive clinical picture which may be a syndrome, i.e., a group of signs or symptoms which cluster together and co-vary over time. Examples are cough, fever and chest pain as seen in pneumonia, or the rapid speech, elevated mood, and psychomotor excitement seen in the manic syndrome. More rarely, the distinctive clinical picture may consist of an isolated sign or symptom in the absence of other signs indicating a more pervasive disorder. Examples are the characteristic pain of *Trigeminal Neuralgia* and simple *Stuttering*. Finally, at the highest level, a specific etiology or pathophysiology is known which accounts for the distinctive clinical picture. This constitutes a disease level of understanding. Examples are *Pneumococcal Pneumonia* and *Amphetamine Schizophreniform Syndrome*.

In DSM-III, as in the rest of medicine, all diagnostic categories are conceptualized at either the distinctive clinical picture or the disease level of comprehension. This is because the first level of comprehension, the isolated sign or symptom without reference to associated features or cause, has very little predictive value.

Most of the DSM-III categories represent distinctive clinical pictures consisting of syndromes (e.g., *Schizophrenic and Affective Disorders*). There are a few DSM-III categories which represent isolated signs or symptoms not explainable by a more pervasive disorder (e.g., *Stuttering* and some of the *Sexual Dysfunctions*). Some of the *Organic Mental Disorders* are described at the disease level (e.g., *Alcohol Amnestic Disorder*).

The term "disorder" has been chosen as the most general term to be applied to all of the conditions listed in DSM-III. This term has been chosen as preferable to alternative terms such as "disease," "illness," or "reaction," each of which would seem to be inappropriate for some of the conditions. Disease would be an appropriate term only for some of the *Organic Mental Disorders,* since only in these conditions has a specific etiology or pathophysiological process been demonstrated. The term "illness" has been used by some to refer only to the active clinical manifestations of an underlying disease in the host (2). Finally, the term "reaction," which was used for most of the conditions in DSM-I, has had a history of varied meanings, most recently to indicate psychosocial causation. (We note that the ICD has no consistent term for the conditions listed; the section dealing with psychiatric conditions is titled, "Mental disorders.")

Within the Medical Model

We regard the medical model as a working hypothesis that there are organismic dysfunctions which are relatively distinct with regard to clinical features, etiology, and course. No assumption is made regarding the primacy of biological over social or environmental etiological factors. In addition, it is assumed that for many medical disorders a single sufficient and necessary cause is unlikely, and that usually what is involved is a complex interaction of biological and environmental events.

There is considerable concern among many mental health professionals that psychiatry inappropriately assumes that the conditions it describes in its official nomenclature represent independent disease entities, clearly separate from one another and from problems of everyday living. Kendell (3) has suggested that before a given diagnostic category can be regarded as a disease *entity*, it is necessary to demonstrate discontinuity between this given category and other categories, and between the given category and normality. He suggests that this is possible when it can be demonstrated that mild forms of the disorder, or inter-forms mixing features of two disorders, are less common than the fully developed or pure form of the disorder. He argues that using this criterion there is no justification for regarding the functional psychiatric disorders as disease entities. However, he also points out that in the rest of medicine there are some established medical disorders which also lack evidence justifying disease entity status. An example is *Essential Hypertension* which is more common in mild than severe forms. The justification for using a categorical approach in DSM-III which treats psychiatric conditions as separate disorders connoting entity status if not denoting it lies in the practical utility of such typology for communication, treatment, and research, despite theoretical limitations. Furthermore, the history of medicine attests to the value of categorical subdivision in the discovery of specific etiology and treatments.

Principles of Organization

Several principles have been used in DSM-III to determine the grouping of individual disorders into classes. In order of priority, they are as follows:

(1) Know necessary organic etiology. This constitutes the foundation for the class of *Organic Mental Disorders* and *Drug Use Disorders*.

(2) Shared phenomenology. This principle includes both cross-sectional clinical picture as well as longitudinal course, and is the basis for the class of *Schizophrenic Disorders, Paranoid Disorders, Affective Disorders, Anxiety Disorders, Somatoform Disorders, Dissociative Disorders, Personality Disorders,* and *Disorders of Impulse Control.*

(3) Known or presumed necessary psychosocial etiology. This is the basis for the class of *Reactive Disorders Not Classified Elsewhere,* and includes the *Adjustment Disorders.*

Because intrapsychic conflict exists in so many psychiatric disorders as well as in persons without psychiatric disorders, it is not used in DSM-III as the basis for class formation, hence the absence of the traditional category, "the neuroses." The psychoanalytic concept of neurosis implies an etiology of conflict resolution by the process of symptom formation, and implies a rough index of illness severity as well. As an etiological concept, the term "neurosis" might be applicable to many disorders included in DSM-III but not included in previous classifications and not usually regarded as traditional neurotic subtypes. Examples would include some *Sexual Dysfunctions,* some cases of *Anorexia Nervosa,* and some cases of *Multiple Personality.* If disorders were grouped together on the basis of intrapsychic conflict and symptom resolution, it is not at all clear what the class boundaries would be.

In determining the sequencing of the classes, the same order of principles is used as in class formation. Thus, the first two classes are the *Organic Mental Disorders* and the *Drug Use Disorders.* In addition, classes are listed in decreasing order of symptomatic comprehensiveness. For example, *Schizophrenic Disorders,* which may include thought disorder and hallucinations, precedes *Paranoid Disorders* which includes neither of these. *Affective Disorders* precedes *Anxiety Disorders* because all of the manifestations of *Anxiety Disorders* can occur in patients with *Affective Disorders,* though the converse is not true.

There are many classes, *Somatoform Disorders, Dissociative Disorders, Personality Disorders, Sexual Disorders,* and *Disorders Usually Arising in Childhood or Adolescence,* for which the sequencing principles do not appear useful, and the order chosen reflects, as much as possible, the sequencing used in ICD-9. The last two specific classes of disorders represent residual categories, *Reactive Disorders Not Classified Elsewhere, Disorders of Impulse Control Not Classified Elsewhere* and *Sleep Disorders.* The ordering and composition of the diagnostic classes are illustrated in the most recent draft of the classification as shown in Table 1.

Multiaxial Approach

The purpose of the multiaxial approach is to insure that certain information of value in predicting outcome and planning treatment are

DRAFT OF AXES I and II of DSM–III CLASSIFICATION* as of March 30, 1977

Note: For multiaxial diagnosis, each patient is coded on each of the five axes.

ORGANIC MENTAL DISORDERS

1. This section includes those organic mental disorders in which the etiology or pathogenesis is listed below (taken from the mental disorders section of ICD-9-CM).

Senile and pre-senile dementias

Code organic mental disorder in fifth digit as 1 = (uncomplicated), 2 = with delirium, 3 = with delusional features, 4 = with depressive features, 9 = unspecified.

290.0x Senile dementia
290.1x Pre-senile dementia
290.4x Repeated infarct dementia

Drug induced

Alcohol
291.60 intoxication
291.40 idiosyncratic intoxication (Pathological intoxication)
291.80 withdrawal
291.00 withdrawal delirium (Delirium tremens)
291.30 withdrawal hallucinosis
291.10 amnestic syndrome (Wernicke-Korsakoff syndrome)
Barbiturate or related acting sedative or hypnotic
292.01 intoxication
292.81 withdrawal syndromes
292.31 amnestic syndrome
Opioid
292.02 intoxication
292.82 withdrawal
Cocaine
292.03 intoxication
Amphetamine or related acting

2. This section includes those organic mental disorders in which the etiology or pathogenesis is either noted as an additional diagnosis from outside of the mental disorders section of ICD-9-CM (Axis III) or is unknown.

293.00 Delirium
294.10 Dementia
294.00 Amnestic syndrome
293.20 Organic delusional syndrome
293.30 Hallucinosis
293.40 Organic affective syndrome
310.10 Organic personality syndrome
294.80 Other or mixed organic brain syndrome
294.90 Unspecified organic brain syndrome

DRUG USE DISORDERS (including alcohol)

Code course of illness in fourth (Alcoholism) or fifth digit as 1 = continuous, 2 = episodic, 3 = in remission, 9 = unspecified.

303.x0 Alcohol dependence (Alcoholism)
305.0x Alcohol abuse
304.1x Barbiturate or related acting sedative or hypnotic dependence
305.4x Barbiturate or related acting sedative or hypnotic abuse
304.0x Opioid dependence
305.5x Opioid abuse
304.2x Cocaine dependence
305.6x Cocaine abuse

AFFECTIVE DISORDERS

Episodic affective disorders

Code severity of episode in fifth digit as .1 = mild, 2 = moderate, 3 = severe but not psychotic, 4 = severe and psychotic, 5 = in partial remission 6 = in full remission, 9 = unspecified.

Manic disorder
296.0x single episode
296.1x recurrent
Depressive disorder
296.2x single episode
296.3x recurrent
Bipolar affective disorder
296.4x manic
296.5x depressed
296.6x mixed

Intermittent affective disorders

301.11 Intermittent depressive disorder (Depressive character)
301.12 Intermittent hypomanic disorder (Hypomanic personality)
301.13 Intermittent bipolar disorder (Cyclothymic personality)

Atypical affective disorders

296.80 Atypical depressive disorder
296.90 Atypical manic disorder
296.70 Atypical bipolar disorder

PSYCHOSES NOT ELSEWHERE CLASSIFIED

298.80 Brief reactive psychosis
298.90 Atypical psychosis

ANXIETY DISORDERS

Phobic Disorders

sympathomimetic
292.04 intoxication
292.14 delirium
292.44 organic delusional syndrome
292.84 withdrawal
Hallucinogen
292.05 intoxication
292.45 organic delusional syndrome
292.65 organic affective syndrome
Cannabis
292.06 intoxication
292.46 organic delusional syndrome
292.76 organic personality syndrome
Tobacco
292.87 withdrawal
Caffeine
292.08 intoxication(caffeinism)
Other, mixed, or unspecified drug
292.09 intoxication
292.19 delirium
292.29 dementia
292.39 amnestic syndrome
292.49 organic delusional syndrome
292.59 hallucinosis
292.69 organic affective syndrome
292.79 organic personality syndrome
292.89 withdrawal
292.99 unspecified organic brain syndrome

304.4x Amphetamine or related acting sympathomimetic dependence
305.7x Amphetamine or related acting sympathomimetic abuse
Hallucinogen
305.3x Hallucinogen abuse
Cannabis
304.3x Cannabis dependence
305.2x Cannabis abuse
305.1x Tobacco use disorder
304.7x Combination of opioid type drug with any other dependence
304.8x Combinations of drug dependence excluding opioid type drug
304.6x Other specified drug dependence
304.9x Unspecified drug dependence
305.9x Other, mixed, or unspecified drug abuse

SCHIZOPHRENIC DISORDERS
Course of illness may be coded in fifth digit as 1 = acute, 2 = subacute, 3 = subchronic, 4 = chronic, 5 = in remission, 9 = unspecified.
295.1x Disorganized (Hebephrenic)
295.2x Catatonic
295.3x Paranoid
295.7x Schizo-affective, depressed
295.8x Schizo-affective, manic
295.9x Undifferentiated
295.6x Residual

PARANOID DISORDERS
297.10 Paranoia
297.30 Shared paranoid disorder (Folie à deux)
297.00 Paranoid state
297.90 Unspecified paranoid disorder

300.21 Agoraphobia with panic attacks
300.22 Agoraphobia without panic attacks
300.23 Social phobia
300.24 Simple phobia
300.29 Unspecified phobia
300.01 Panic disorder
300.30 Obsessive compulsive disorder
300.02 Generalized anxiety disorder
300.09 Atypical anxiety disorder

FACTITIOUS DISORDERS
300.15 Factitious illness with psychological symptoms
300.16 Chronic factitious illness with physical symptoms (Munchausen syndrome)
300.17 Other factitious illness with physical symptoms
300.18 Unspecified factitious illness

SOMATOFORM DISORDERS
300.81 Somatization disorder (Briquet's disorder)
300.11 Conversion disorder
307.80 Psychalgia
300.70 Atypical somatoform disorder

DISSOCIATIVE DISORDERS
300.12 Amnesia
300.13 Fugue
300.14 Multiple personality
300.60 Depersonalization
300.19 Other or unspecified

*Note: The traditional neurotic subtypes are included in the Affective, Anxiety, Somatoform, and Dissociative Disorders.

PERSONALITY DISORDERS
Note. These are coded on Axis II.

301.00 Paranoid
301.20 Asocial (Schizoid)
295.50 Schizotypal (Latent, Borderline schizophrenia)

301.50 Histrionic
301.81 Narcissistic
301.70 Antisocial
301.83 Unstable (Borderline personality organization)

301.82 Avoidant
301.60 Dependent
301.40 Compulsive

301.88 Other, mixed, or unspecified

PSYCHOSEXUAL DISORDERS
Gender identity or role disorders
Indicate sexual history in the fifth digit of Transsexualism code as 1 = asexual, 2 = homosexual, 3 = heterosexual, 4 = mixed, 9 = unspecified.

302.5x Transsexualism
302.30 Transvestism
302.61 Gender identity or role disorder of childhood
302.62 Other gender identity or role disorders of adult life

Paraphilias
302.81 Fetishism
302.10 Zoophilia
302.20 Pedophilia
302.00 Dyshomophilia
302.40 Exhibitionism
302.82 Voyeurism
302.83 Sexual masochism

Pervasive developmental disorders
299.00 Infantile autism
299.80 Early childhood psychosis
299.20 Pervasive developmental disorder of childhood, residual state
299.90 Unspecified

Attention deficit disorders
314.00 with hyperactivity
314.10 without hyperactivity

Specific developmental disorders
Note: These are coded on Axis II.
315.00 Specific reading disorder
315.10 Specific arithmetical disorder
315.30 Developmental language disorder
315.40 Developmental articulation disorder
315.50 Coordination disorder
Indicate course in the fifth digit as 1 = primary, 2 = secondary, 9 = unspecified.
307.6x Enuresis
307.7x Encopresis
315.80 Mixed
315.90 Other
Unspecified

Stereotyped movement disorders
307.21 Motor tic disorder
307.22 Motor-verbal tic disorder (Gilles de la Tourette)
307.29 Unspecified tic disorder
307.30 Other

Speech disorders not elsewhere classified
307.00 Stuttering
307.91 Elective mutism

Conduct disorders
Code severity in fifth digit as 1 = mild, 2 = moderate, 3 = severe, 9 = unspecified.
312.0x Undersocialized conduct disorder,

DISORDERS OF IMPULSE CONTROL NOT ELSEWHERE CLASSIFIED
312.31 Pathological gambling
312.32 Kleptomania
312.33 Pyromania
312.34 Intermittent explosive disorder
312.35 Isolated explosive disorder
312.38 Other- or unspecified impulse control disorder

SLEEP DISORDERS
Non-organic
307.41 Temporary insomnia
307.42 Persistent insomnia
307.43 Temporary hypersomnia
307.44 Persistent hypersomnia
307.45 Non-organic sleep-wake cycle disturbance
307.46 Somnambulism
307.47 Night terrors
307.48 Other non-organic dyssomnias
307.49 Unspecified non-organic sleep disorder

Organic
780.51 Insomnia associated with diseases elsewhere classified
780.52 Insomnia with central sleep-apnea
780.53 Other organic insomnia
780.54 Hypersomnia associated with diseases elsewhere classified
780.55 Hypersomnia associated with obstructive or mixed sleep-apnea
780.56 Other organic hypersomnia
780.57 Organic sleep-wake cycle disturbance
780.58 Organic dyssomnias
780.59 Unspecified organic sleep disorder

OTHER DISORDERS AND CONDITIONS
Unspecified mental disorder (non-psychotic)

302.84 Sexual sadism
302.85 Other

Psychosexual dysfunctions
302.71 with inhibited sexual desire
302.72 with inhibited sexual excitement (frigidity, impotence)
302.73 with inhibited female orgasm
302.74 with inhibited male orgasm
302.75 with premature ejaculation
302.76 with functional dyspareunia
302.77 with functional vaginismus
302.78 other
302.79 unspecified

Other psychosexual disorders
302.90 Psychosexual disorder not elsewhere classified

DISORDERS USUALLY ARISING IN CHILDHOOD OR ADOLESCENCE
This section lists conditions that usually manifest themselves in childhood or adolescence. However, any appropriate adult diagnosis can be used for diagnosing a child.

Mental retardation
Code a 1 in the fifth digit to indicate association with a known biological factor which must be coded on Axis III. Otherwise code 0.
317.0x Mild mental retardation
318.0x Moderate mental retardation
318.1x Severe mental retardation
318.2x Profound mental retardation
319.0x Unspecified mental retardation

aggressive type
312.1x Undersocialized conduct disorder, unaggressive type
312.2x Socialized conduct disorder

Eating disorders
307.10 Anorexia nervosa
307.51 Bulimia
307.52 Pica
307.53 Rumination
307.58 Other or unspecified

Anxiety disorders of childhood or adolescence
309.21 Separation anxiety disorder
313.20 Shyness disorder
313.00 Overanxious disorder

Disorders characteristic of late adolescence
309.22 Emancipation disorder of adolescence or early adult life
313.60 Identity disorder
309.23 Specific academic or work inhibition

Other disorders of childhood or adolescence
313.50 Oppositional disorder
313.70 Academic underachievement disorder

REACTIVE DISORDERS NOT ELSEWHERE CLASSIFIED
309.81 Post traumatic disorder

Adjustment disorders
300.40 with depressed mood
309.28 with anxious mood
309.24 with mixed emotional features
309.82 with physical symptoms
309.30 with disturbance of conduct
309.40 with mixed disturbance of emotions and conduct
309.83 with withdrawal
309.90 other or unspecified

307.99 Unspecified mental disorder (non-psychotic)

Psychic factors in physical condition
Specify physical condition on Axis III and degree of psychological component in the fourth digit as 1 = probable, 2 = prominent, 3 = unknown or unspecified degree.
316.x0 Psychic factors in physical condition

No mental disorder
V71.00 No mental disorder

Conditions not attributable to a known mental disorder
V65.20 Malingering
V71.01 Adult antisocial behavior
V71.02 Childhood or adolescent antisocial behavior
V61.10 Marital problem
V61.20 Parent-child problem
V62.81 Other interpersonal problem
V62.20 Occupational problem
V62.82 Simple bereavement
V15.81 Noncompliance with medical treatment
V62.88 Other life circumstance problem

Administrative categories
799.90 Diagnosis deferred
V70.70 Research subject
V63.20 Boarder
V68.30 Referral without need for evaluation

recorded for each patient (8). This is done by recording these classes of information on each of five axes. The first and second axes are used to record the mental disorders, with the second axis specifically reversed for *Personality Disorders* in adults, and *Specific Developmental Disorders* in children. These latter conditions tend to be ignored while attention is focused on the acute clinical disturbance. Within axis 11 there are categories which may have to be used when either *Personality Disorder* or *Specific Developmental Disorder* does not exist, cannot be identified, or appears to be the persistent residue of a major mental disorder (e.g., schizoid features and reduced spontaneity following an episode of *Schizophrenic Disorder*).

Axis III is reserved for listing non-mental medical disorders that are judged to be pertinent to the etiology or management of the psychiatric disorder listed on axes I and II. These conditions are taken from the non-mental disorder chapters from ICD-9. An example of *Renal Insufficiency* (affecting use of Lithium Carbonate) coded on axis III with *Bipolar Affective Disorder* coded on axis I. Another example is *Pneumonia* coded on axis III judged to be of etiologic importance to a *Delirium* noted on axis I.

Axis IV permits the clinician to indicate the severity of one or more psychosocial stressors which are judged likely to have contributed to the development or exacerbation of the current episode of mental disorder which is coded on axis I.

The rating of severity of stress should be based on the clinician's assessment of the stress or change in usual life patterns that an average person would experience from the event or events. The number of stressful events, their duration, and the context in which they occur should be taken into account, including the degree to which the event is desired and is under the individual's control. However, the patient's idiosyncratic vulnerability or reaction should not influence the rating. In most instances, the psychosocial stressor will have occurred within the year prior to the current episode of illness (*Post Traumatic Disorder* is a notable exception). Frequently, the psychosocial stressor may itself be in part a consequence of the individual's psychopathology—for example, Alcoholism leading to marital difficulties, eventuating in a divorce, which then is a psychosocial stressor contributing to the development of a superimposed Depressive Disorder.

Physical events, such as illness, or accidents, should be evaluated on this Axis on the basis of the psychological impact of such events.

The following codes and terms should be used:

Code	Term	Definition or Examples
1	None	No apparent psychosocial stressor
2	Minimal	Vacation, minor violations of the law, small bank loan
3	Mild	Began or ended school, argument with neighbor or boss, change in work hours
4	Moderate	Change to different line of work, death of close friend, pregnancy, child leaves home
5	Severe	Severe illness in self or family, bankruptcy, marital separation, birth of child
6	Extreme	Death of close relative, divorce, jail term
7	Catastrophic	Multiple family death, concentration camp experience, devastating natural disaster
9	Unspecified	No information or not applicable

Information on axis IV should be recorded in the following manner:

IV Psychosocial stressors: 5 Severe (Business failure)

For special purposes, the type of psychosocial stressor may be coded using the classification included in the appendix.

Axis V permits the clinician to indicate the highest level of adaptive functioning exhibited by the patient during the past year. This information will frequently have prognostic implications that will be of value in formulating a comprehensive treatment plan.

The clinician should indicate the highest overall level of adaptive functioning that was characteristic of the patient for at least a few months during the past year, taking into account routine and expected activities, such as role performance (as a worker, student, housekeeper, parent, etc.), social functioning, self-care, and the absence of any self-imposed restrictions on autonomy. This axis reflects the level of adaptive functioning and not subjective distress or other psychopathological signs or symptoms.

The following codes and terms should be used:

Code	Term	Definition or Examples
1	Superior	Unusually effective functioning in a wide range of activities and relationships
2	Very good	Better than average functioning in many activities and relationships without any significant impairment in any area
3	Good	Adequate in almost all areas and no more than slight impairment in any area
4	Fair	Generally functioning adequately but some impairment in at least one area
5	Poor	Marked impairment in several areas of functioning
6	Very poor	Major impairment in most areas of functioning
7	Grossly impaired	Unable to function in almost all areas
9	Unspecified	No information or not applicable

Information on axis V should be recorded in the following manner:

V Highest level of adaptive functioning past year: 4 Fair

We have resisted the temptation to add still further axes, such as current severity of functional impairment, and course. (It should be noted that for several of the classes of disorders, additional dimensions are included within the coding of axis I at the fourth or fifth digit level. For example, the phenomenology of the current episode of *Schizophrenic Disorders* is noted in the fourth digit, and the course in the fifth digit. Another example is the inclusion of the severity dimension of *Affective Disorders* in the fifth digit.) Although axes I, II and III previously have been integrated into traditional comprehensive diagnosis, axes IV and V have been added because of their importance and simplicity in providing information relevant to etiology, management and long-term outcome. Multiaxial diagnosis should be an improvement over traditional psychiatric diagnosis, but is in no way a substitute for a comprehensive case formulation. Conceptually, multiaxial diagnosis represents an advance in breadth and flexibility. Only use will determine if it is feasible in varied clinical settings.

Operational Criteria

Central among the innovations in DSM-III is the use of suggested operational criteria for each diagnostic category. In DSM-I and II, as well as in ICD-8 and 9, the clinician is to a large degree on his own in defining the content and boundaries of the diagnostic categories, since explicit detailed definitions are not provided (7). To remedy this dilemma, a number of diagnostic schemes in psychiatry have employed operational definitions which involve the use of specific inclusion and exclusion criteria for each diagnosis. With this approach, the clinician's task is twofold: to determine the presence or absence of specific clinical phenomena, and then to apply the comprehensive rules provided for making the diagnosis. This approach was first developed by the St. Louis group, and is often referred to as the "Feighner criteria" because Feighner was the senior author of a paper summarizing their criteria for 15 conditions (1). As part of a collaborative project on the psychobiology of the depressive disorders sponsored by the Clinical Research Branch of the NIMH, Spitzer, Endicott and Robins expanded and modified the Feighner criteria for a selected group of 23 functional disorders, and demonstrated that their use greatly increased interrater reliability (7). This new set of criteria, the *Research Diagnostic Criteria* (RDC), has been further modified and included in the operational criteria for DSM-III. Furthermore, it has been a model for the development of the operational criteria for the large number of categories in DSM-III not represented in the RDC. Table 2 illustrates the use of operational criteria for the DSM-III diagnosis of a depressive episode.

In research settings, it is important to minimize false positives since the purpose is to study homogenous subgroups. On the other hand, in clinical settings it is important to minimize false negatives which would deprive patients of needed treatment. Therefore, unlike the RDC and the Feighner criteria, a diagnosis can be made in DSM-III when the clinician does not have sufficient information to be certain that the patient satisfies the full criteria, though it appears clinically probable. An example might be a patient satisfying the symptomatic criteria for *Schizophrenic Disorder* but for whom no information is available on duration of present illness. In the presence of clinical features which suggest a chronic illness, such as flat affect, the physician would be justified in concluding that in all likelihood the patient does satisfy the full operational criteria.

Reliability and Face Validity Precede Predictive Validity

We recognize that many of the newer as well as traditional categories in DSM-III have insufficient evidence of predictive validity in the sense

TABLE 2

Operational Criteria for an Episode of Depressive Disorder

A. Dysphoric mood or pervasive loss of interest. The disturbance is characterized by symptoms such as the following: depressed, sad, blue, hopeless, low, down in the dumps, "don't care anymore," irritable, worried. The disturbance must be prominent and relatively persistent but not necessarily the most dominant symptom. It does not include momentary shifts from one dysphoric mood to another dysphoric mood, e.g., anxiety to depression to anger, such as are seen in states of acute psychotic turmoil.

B. At least four of the following symptoms:
   (1) Poor appetite or weight loss or increased appetite or weight gain (change of one lb. a week or ten lbs. a year when not dieting).
   (2) Sleep difficulty or sleeping too much.
   (3) Loss of energy, fatigability, or tiredness.
   (4) Psychomotor agitation or retardation (but not mere subjective feelings of restlessness or being slowed down).
   (5) Loss of interest or pleasure in usual activities, or decrease in sexual drive (do not include if limited to a period when delusional or hallucinating).
   (6) Feelings of self-reproach or excessive or inappropriate guilt (either may be delusional).
   (7) Complaints or evidence of diminished ability to think or concentrate such as slow thinking, or indecisiveness (do not include if associated with obvious formal thought disorder).
   (8) Recurrent thoughts of death or suicide, including thoughts of wishing to be dead.

C. The period of illness has had a duration of at least 1 week from the time of the first noticeable change in the patient's usual condition.

D. None of the following which suggests Schizophrenia is present:
   (1) Delusions of being controlled or thought broadcasting, insertion, or withdrawal.
   (2) Hallucinations of any type throughout the day for several days or intermittently throughout a one-week period unless all of the content is clearly related to depression or elation.
   (3) Auditory hallucinations in which either a voice keeps up a running commentary on the patient's behaviors or thoughts as they occur, or two or more voices converse with each other.
   (4) At some time during the period of illness had delusions or hallucinations for more than one month in the absence of prominent affective (manic or depressive) symptoms (although typical depressive delusions, such as delusions of guilt, sin, poverty, nihilism, or self-deprecation or hallucinations with similar content are permitted).
   (5) Preoccupation with a delusion or hallucination to the relative exclusion of other symptoms or concerns (other than delusions of guilt, sin, poverty, nihilism, or self-deprecation, or hallucinations with similar content).
   (6) Marked formal thought disorder if accompanied by either blunted or inappropriate affect, delusions or hallucinations of any type, or grossly disorganized 'behavior.

E. Not due to any specific known Organic Mental Disorder.

F. Not superimposed on Schizophrenia, Residual Subtype.

G. Excludes Simple Bereavement following loss of a loved one if all of the features are commonly seen in members of the subject's subcultural group in similar circumstances.

of providing useful information for treatment assignment or outcome. By providing operational definitions of the disorders that will permit family, treatment and outcome studies, as well as systematic inquiry into etiology, the ultimate predictive validity of the DSM-III diagnoses can be determined with an accuracy heretofore impossible. This will result in the refinement of some categories, the elimination of others, and the probable addition of entirely new categories.

Systematic and Comprehensive Description of the Disorders

Traditional glossaries accompanying national or international classifications generally describe in an unsystematic manner only the most characteristic features of the disorders. The text of DSM-III systematically describes each disorder in terms of current knowledge in the following areas: essential features (those features that must be present for the diagnosis to be made), associated features (those features frequently but not always present), and, when known, usual age at onset, course, predisposing factors, impairment, complications, prevalence, familial pattern, sex ratio, and differential diagnosis.

For many of the disorders that have been carefully studied, such as the *Schizophrenic* and *Affective Disorders,* the descriptions are quite extensive. Consequently, DSM-III will be a much larger document than its predecessors or the ICD-9 glossary and there may be a need for a version to be used in certain settings which summarizes the material.

Compatibility with ICD-9 at the Four Digit Level

The DSM-III disorders will utilize five digit codes. The first four of these are identical to the closest corresponding ICD-9 category. The fifth digit permits greater specification and flexibility in the DSM-III system. For example, the DSM-III code for *Depressive Disorder, Recurrent, Psychotic,* is 296.34. The first four digits correspond to the ICD-9 category of *Manic depressive psychosis, depressed type.*

Frequently, the DSM-III names for the disorders have been changed from ICD-9 and traditional usage. This has been done only when the Task Force became convinced that the accumulated connotations of the ICD-9 or traditional term were sufficiently misleading as to warrant use of fresh and simple language. For example, the ICD-9 term of *Manic depressive psychosis, depressed type,* to describe a disorder characterized by recurrent depressions implies that the disorder is part of a larger psychotic condition which includes both manic and depressive features. As evidence has accumulated to suggest that this is not the case, the term *Depressive Disorder, Recurrent,* seemed more accurate and preferable. In a similar vein, the research diagnosis of *Unipolar Depression* was considered for this disorder but rejected after discussion revealed the connotation of a purely biological etiology. On the other hand, the term *Bipolar Affective Disorder* was retained because it provided the best accurate description and was not a source of controversy despite its origins in biological psychiatry.

Deviations from ICD-9 are not limited to additional digits and changes in some names. Because of the principles involved in grouping disorders into classes and sequencing the classes in the listing, the order of the categories in DSM-III departs widely from ICD-9, and this accounts for the lack of sequential order in the code numbers attached to the DSM-III disorders.

The Task Force has had to weigh the assets of departing from ICD-9 against the liabilities. These include difficulties in communicating with our psychiatric colleagues in other nations, and potential incompatibility in diagnostic information accumulated by national health registers. We believe that the innovations in DSM-III leading to greater accuracy and validation of psychiatric diagnosis justify the departures from ICD-9 that have been made.

Field Testing Prior to Official Adoption

In a sense, the wide exposure of draft versions of DSM-III to the profession has constituted the first field trial of DSM-III. There is no class of disorders in DSM-III that has not been extensively revised, in some cases over 20 times, before a satisfactory, though untested, version has emerged. Current plans for the immediate further refinement of DSM-III consist of national field trials at a large number of representative facilities and in private offices as well.

The purpose of this field testing is to eliminate as many problems as possible before the final draft of the manual is published, and to provide answers to the following questions:

1. Which diagnostic terms cannot be applied readily?

2. What are the ambiguities in the diagnostic criteria, if any?

3. What are the conditions for which DSM-III does not provide a diagnostic category?

4. What problems does the new nomenclature present in coding diagnostic terms for data processing and administrative review?

5. To what extent are DSM-III and ICD-9 categories compatible?

The field studies are planned in two phases. During the first phase, only portions of the DSM-III will be applied to patients at a given facility. Thus, only the categories of *Schizophrenic, Paranoid, Affective* and *Anxiety Disorders* will be tested with patients in general inpatient and outpatient facilities. The *Organic Mental Disorders* will be tested in liaison services within general hospitals and specialized services for geriatric patients. The *Sexual Disorders* will be studied in specialized clinics for the treatment of sexual dysfunctions and gender role disturbances. The *Drug Use Disorders* will be studied in substance abuse clinics and inpatient drug and alcohol programs. The *Child and Adolescent Disorders* will be studied in child psychiatry clinics and inpatient services and in college mental health services. The *Personality Disorders* will be studied in outpatient clinics and private practice settings. Phase two will involve testing of the entire manual with a focus on multiaxial diagnosis. In both phases, the information received will be used to modify the diagnostic descriptions, operational criteria, and instructions for use.

CONCLUSION

DSM-III is the first national classification system in psychiatry to utilize operational criteria, explicit principles of classification, a multiaxial approach to diagnosis, and extensive field testing prior to official adoption. Although to some the work of the Task Force seems radical · and mistaken (8), we believe that the principles that are guiding the development of DSM-III will prove fruitful for both the scientific and clinical development of psychiatry.

Appendix
CLASSIFICATION OF PSYCHOLOGICAL STRESSORS
GLOSSARY OF TERMS

01 No significant distortion of psychosocial environment
Stresses and adversities of mild degree only (as well as a fully normal psychosocial environment) would be coded here.

I. *Familial Setting*

02 *Mental disturbance in other family member(s)*

Any kind of overt, handicapping psychiatric disorder or any kind of *gross* abnormality of behavior (*not* necessarily receiving psychiatric treatment) in a member of the patient's immediate household or in a spouse, child, parent or sib of the patient regardless of whether or not they are in the same household.

03 *Physical illness in other family member(s)*

Any kind of overt, serious, or handicapping disorder diagnosed or suspected in a member of the patient's immediate household or in a spouse, child, parent or sib of the patient regardless of whether or not they are in the same household.

04 *Discordant intra-familial relationships*

Discord or disharmony (such as shown by hostility, quarrelling, scapegoating, etc.) of sufficient severity to lead to a persisting atmosphere in the home or to persisting interpersonal tensions. Discordant relationships between spouse and patient, child and patient, parent and patient and discordant relationships with a sib or any immediate family member should be included here (irrespective of whether they are living together).

05 *Lack of warmth in family or parenting person(s), including institutional*

A *marked* lack of warmth or affection; or a coldness and distance in the relationships between the parents or between parent and patient (irrespective of whether they are living together); lack of empathetic responsiveness as distinct from punitiveness or restrictiveness.

06 *Familial over-involvement*

A *marked* excess of intrusiveness (such as shown by over-protection, over-restriction, incestuous relationships or undue emotional stimulation, etc.) by another family member when judged in relation to the patient's maturity level and the socio-familial context.

07 *Inadequate or distorted intra-familial communications*

A *marked* lack or distortion of communication or discussion between family members of such severity that important family issues are either not discussed or are the subject of misleading messages between family members.

08 *Inadequate or inconsistent parental control*

A *marked* lack of effective control or supervision of the patient's activities when judged in relation to the patient's maturity level and the socio-familial context. Markedly inconsistent or inefficient discipline should be coded here.

09 Inadequate social, linguistic or perceptual stimulation

A *marked* lack of effective and meaningful social, linguistic *or* perceptual experiences when judged in relation to the patient's developmental needs, whether arising as a result of inadequate or inappropriate parent-child interaction, periods of poor quality substitute care, or for any other reason. A marked lack of toys, a failure to engage the child in adequate play or conversation, or a gross isolation from other children would all be included. An institutional upbringing which provided adequate cognitive stimulation but a marked lack of affective ties should also be coded here.

10 Other intra-familial psychosocial stress

Any recent or current *marked* stress on the patient arising within the family such as caused by bereavement, divorce, or separation; the departure of a loved person from within the home, or the addition of a new member.

II. *Individual — Likely to Be Limited to Patient in Effect*

11 Crime

Psychological reaction to being a victim of a crime against person or property.

12 Accused of or prosecuted for a crime or alleged wrongdoing

Psychological reaction to prosecution for a criminal act and allegations of criminal and non-criminal but morally reprehensible actions.

13 Child abuse—physical and psychological

Beatings, torturing, starving and extreme verbal attacks or unremitting criticism.

14 Sexual abuse

Rape; other sexual molestation with or without battery. The issue of consent is relevant only to adults.

15 Psychological reaction to physical illness, including the threat of death or functional disability

Accident, pregnancy, abortion, female or male menopause.

16 Financial problems

Inadequate finances, where the amount of money available is insufficient to cover the necessary expenses, e.g., rent, food, medical expenses, clothing.

17 School or work environment stresses

Loss of job or no job, inability to cope with the work involved, marked instability in the school or work environment, or increased responsibility.

18 *Other extra-familial interpersonal stress*

Any recent or current *marked* stress on the patient arising outside the family such as caused by bereavement, broken important relationship, personal rejection.

19 *Social isolation*

Severe, a person who has little or no contact, less than three contacts per week, either in face to face meetings or by telephone, with family, friends and neighbors; moderate, doesn't have regular contacts to depend on in an emergency, has few accessible friends, and is not friendly with his neighbors.

III. *Community — Likely to Occur in a Group Setting or Involve Many Others*

20 *Natural disaster*

Any recent disaster impinging on the patient which arises as a result of natural causes which leads to severe social disruption or social disadvantage. Floods, earthquakes, volcanoes, landslides, damage due to storm would all be included.

21 *Mass catastrophe as a result of human intent, error or accident*

Civilian victim of warfare, hostage or terrorists not selected by group membership, airplane, train, bus crashes, fires.

22 *Physical environment*

Any stress due to a change in the physical environment in which the stress is not apparent primarily due to a change in interpersonal relationships. Includes moving, home alterations, home repairs, disruption of regularly used utility services, disruption of regularly used travel services.

23 *Military experience and combat*

Military personnel only, reaction to the stresses of training, combat, prisoner of war situations, including brainwashing, and military personnel if treated as concentration camp inmates.

24 *Persecution or adverse discrimination*

Any kind of persecution or gross adverse discrimination on the basis of racial, social, religious, political or other group characteristics which directly impinge on the patient. This includes concentration camp experience.

25 Institutionalization

Any stress due to loss of freedom, difficulty adjusting to new regulations and routines affecting diet, leisure time or mandatory activities, time of awakening or retiring which is associated with entering or being housed in an institutional setting; includes entry into hospital, nursing home, boarding school, prison, religious training center, e.g., monastery, convent, commune.

26 Culture change

Recent migration or movement of the patient to a different socio-cultural environment, or any kind of move which results in a severe disruption of personal ties or relationships (such as eviction resulting in breakup of family or homelessness), or migration of individuals from another socio-cultural environment into his neighborhood.

27 Inadequate living conditions

Grossly inadequate living conditions, however caused. Marked poverty, lack of basic household amenities (bath, hot running water, etc.), overcrowding (to the extent of at least 1-5 persons per all rooms used for living, dining or sleeping), shared beds, vermin infestation of home, and severe damp would all be included.

28 Living in a high crime or delinquency area

Teenagers encouraged to form street gangs, traffic in drugs. Threat of violence to property or person if extortion not paid by individual, Fear of safety at home, in streets, after dark.

IV. Other Categories

88 Other

Any acute or chronic stress, distortion, or disadvantage in a person's psychosocial environments which is not codable above.

98 No psychosocial stressor identified

Despite knowledge of the psychosocial situation surrounding the development of the illness, no stressor has been identified as contributory. This does not mean that there are no psychosocial stressors, but merely that none has ben idetnified.

99 No or inadequate information available on psychological stressors

Patient too disturbed to provide information, and no family member able to supply information.

REFERENCES

1. Feighner, J. P., Robbins, E., Guze, S. B., et al. Diagnostic criteria for use in psychiatric research. *Archives of General Psychiatry*, 1972, 26, 57-63.

2. Feinstein, A. R. *Clinical Judgment.* Baltimore: Williams & Williams, 1967.
3. Kendell, R. W. *The Role of Diagnosis in Psychiatry.* London, England: Blackwell Scientific, 1975.
4. Klein, D. R., & Davis, J. F. *Diagnosis and Drug Treatment of Psychiatric Disorders.* Baltimore: Williams & Williams, 1969.
5. Schimel, J. L. The retreat from a psychiatry of people. *Journal of the American Academy of Psychoanalysis* (editorial), April 1976, Vol. 2, pp. 131-153.
6. Spitzer, R. L., & Endicott, J. *Proposed Definition of Medical and Mental Disorder for DSM-III.* Presented at annual meeting American Psychiatric Association, Anaheim, California, May 1976.
7. Spitzer, R. L., Endicott, J., & Robbins, E. Clinical criteria for psychiatric diagnosis and DSM-III. *American Journal Psychiatry*, 132:11, pp. 1187-1192.
8. Strauss, J. A comprehensive approach to psychiatric diagnosis. *American Journal of Psychiatry*, November 1975, 132:11, pp. 1193-1197.

2

Psychoanalytic Diagnosis

ROBERT J. STOLLER, M.D.

I: PROBLEMS WITH PSYCHODYNAMICS

Introduction

Although Freud had views regarding diagnosis that did not age well, we should recognize that our psychiatric diagnoses would be quite different without their psychoanalytic history and underpinnings. In addition, certain fundamentals of psychoanalytic thinking, I believe, will some day again make their contribution. In this paper, I shall review that history to find its strengths and flaws and then suggest what aspects I think we should retain.

At the outset, let us recall that the word "diagnosis" has two different meanings: The first is the process of detection one undertakes, and the second is the product of that process; both are called diagnosis. One should also distinguish diagnosis from nomenclature (names, a process of labeling) and classification (an arrangement according to a plan, not necessarily the one we should use for diagnosis). Diagnosis refers to a more complete process than does nomenclature or classification and serves as a very condensed statement—shorthand—for a constellation of data. In psychiatry, it functions as a signifier of the sum of our knowledge about a mental state, aiming to give the most information in the shortest form.

25

To make a proper diagnosis in any branch of medicine there should be: 1) *a syndrome*—a constellation of signs and symptoms common to a group and apparent to an observer; 2) *underlying dynamics (pathogenesis)*—pathophysiology in the rest of medicine; neuropathophysiology, or psychodynamics in psychiatry; 3) *etiology*—those factors from which the dynamics originate. The validity of a diagnosis is confirmed when, in using it, one also implies what the course of the condition and effects of specific treatments will be. Using the term "diagnosis" in this proper sense (3), we can see how far psychiatric diagnosis has to progress before many of its categories fulfill these admirable criteria.

For psychiatric diagnosis is at present sickly, and if this pains us, we can take some comfort in knowing that our reaction accurately marks the flawed nature of our knowledge. But we must not fool ourselves; tinkering will not solve much. Accuracy must await further studies on the processes that energize the behavior we label with a diagnosis.

We all know our nosology works best where the conditions listed— the organic brain disorders—are like those in the rest of medicine. The farther we move from that standard, however, the more confused we become. And the area of greatest weakness is just where psychoanalytic thinking, by its nature, is most involved—the conditions that are the product of desire, of motivation, of choice. These are the personality disorders and their offshoots, the neuroses. This is the very area that most separates psychiatric diagnosis from the rest of medicine. (For simplicity, let us restrict this discussion to the personality disorders.)

Our understanding of underlying dynamics and of etiologies is meager in many areas of psychiatric diagnosis; it is oppressive to know we do not yet have a consensus about what we shall elevate to the status of syndromes. The most troubling instance: We cannot agree what is schizophrenia, or even if there is any such thing or group of things with enough in common that they can be ordered within a single label. And the suggestions that character disorders do not exist as such, or cannot be characterized as they are at present, or have nothing to do with medicine and its diagnoses can find adherents.

We should also confess that there is little organization to our diagnostic "system," except when diagnosing organic brain disease. For the rest of the categories, however, we fall back on techniques that have little in common with each other. At times, we formalize a condition with a label because we think we have delineated a syndrome, that is, an organization of signs and symptoms (e.g., schizophrenia). At other times the reason for the label is nothing more than an outstanding sign (e.g., fetishism), or an outstanding symptom (anxiety neurosis), or a single sign (e.g., enuresis), or a single symptom (e.g., tic), or a chronic way of life (e.g., schizoid personality), or body-organ pathology due in part to mental states (e.g., psychophysiological skin disorder), or drug dependence (e.g., alcohol addiction), or a potpourri with no ruling concept (e.g., marital maladjustment).

This is not our fault, but it is hard to defend such mucking about. Still this is a creative difficulty in that it mirrors our uncertainties and the directions psychiatric research into the causes of treatment of mental states can take.

Psychoanalytic Diagnoses

Let us, by reviewing the attitudes analysts have had in regard to diagnosing, focus now on the issues to be faced when psychodynamic thinking is introduced into the process of diagnosis, and let us also look at the diagnoses analysts have created.

Freud's approach to the subject took the direction analysts have since followed: Interest in surface phenomena gives way to the study of underlying mechanisms.

> The classifications which Freud proposed were based primarily on etiology and not simply on symptomatology. . . . It is important to emphasize this fact for the reason that even today the usual psychiatric classification of mental disorders which are not the consequence of disease or injury of the central nervous system is on the basis of their symptomatology. These are what are known as descriptive classifications and in psychiatry as in any other branch of medicine, descriptive classifications of diseases or disorders are of relatively little value, since proper treatment depends on a knowledge of the *cause* of the symptoms rather than of their nature, and the same symptoms in two different patients may have quite different causes. It is therefore worth while noting that from the very early years of his work with mentally ill patients Freud attempted to go beyond a purely descriptive classification and to set up categories of mental disorders which resembled one another in having a common cause, or, at the very least, a common, underlying, mental mechanism. Moreover, an interest in etiology and in psychopathology, rather than merely in descriptive symptomatology, has continued to characterize the psychoanalytic theory of mental disorders to the present time (1, p. 188).

Although a true diagnosis requires that one still keep an eye on the signs and symptoms, most analysts replace labeling with a fascination for underlying psychodynamics. But the study of psychodynamics is especially one of unconscious processes, and so, from the start, we are rather removed from that *sine qua non* for rational diagnosis, i.e., direct observation. That is the dilemma. A diagnosis is built on sand if not supported by dynamics and etiology, but so is a diagnosis that uses unconfirmed—worse, unconfirmable—dynamics and etiologies.

To see the danger in concentrating on dynamics divorced from indepth observation, we can look now at Freud's diagnostic system, shopworn but not yet repudiated by psychoanalysis.* (Before scoffing, those insisting that genetics or behavioristic systems do better would do well to check the gap between their theories and the observations that can actually be made on patients.) Do not fail to note, despite the quaintness we nowadays sense, the commitment to rational diagnosis, the anchor of which is the attempt to describe the forces that produce the observed signs and symptoms.

Ignoring the organic brain syndromes, not usually the province of psychoanalysts, Freud divides mental conditions into three categories. (I retain here the analytic vocabulary such as "ego" and "libido," though personally not enjoying the jargon.) These are:

1) The *traumatic neuroses,* which result from sudden flooding of the ego by stimuli.

2) The *actual neuroses,* which are caused by libido damming up. Over the years, Freud described three subcategories. The first is neurasthenia, "characterized by feeling of physical tiredness, intracranial pressure, dyspepsia, constipation, spinal paraesthesias and the impoverishment of sexual activity. He . . . sought its aetiology in a type of sexual functioning incapable of adequately discharging libidinal tension (masturbation)" (4, p. 265). The second is anxiety neurosis (as he used the term, not our present usage). He distinguished anxiety neurosis "symptomatically speaking, from *neurasthenia,* because the predominance here of anxiety (chronic anxious expectation; attacks of anxiety or of its somatic equivalents)" (4, p. 38). "In anxiety neurosis, [the] precipitating cause is considered to be the non-discharge of sexual excitation [the accumulation

---

* Although the following review may be tedious, I give Freud's classification at length so that it can be seen as a whole. Doing so at this late date, I indulge the fantasy that—as has not yet quite occurred—it can finally be discarded even by analysts.

of sexual tension, as by abstinence or *coitus interruptus*], while in neurasthenia it is the incomplete satisfaction of it, as in masturbation" (4,
p. 10). The third was hypochondria.

3) The *psychoneuroses* (at first called the neuro-psychoses), the major
category. This term, idiosyncratic by our present standards, includes both
those states we today call neuroses and the "functional" psychoses; its
implication is that its symptoms "are the symbolic expression of infantile
conflicts" (4, p. 369). Freud divided the psychoneuroses into transference
neuroses and narcissistic neuroses. "In contrast to the narcissistic neuroses,
the transference neuroses are characterized by the libido's always being
displaced on to real or imaginary objects instead of being withdrawn
from these and directed on to the ego" (4, p. 462). We use the term
"psychosis" for what Freud called "narcissistic neurosis" (though one
should note that Freud ended by restricting the term "narcissistic neurosis" to melancholia). Narcissistic neurosis is "characterized by the withdrawal of libido from the outside world and its direction on to the ego"
(4, p. 258). The narcissistic neuroses are our "functional" psychoses;
those specifically mentioned by Freud are paranoia, schizophrenia, and
the manic-depressive continuum.

Freud described three types of transference neurosis. The first, anxiety
hysteria (not the same as his term "anxiety neurosis"), is a diagnosis
"introduced by Freud to distinguish a neurosis whose central symptoms
is phobia, and to emphasize its structural resemblance to conversion
hysteria" (4, p. 37). The second, conversion hysteria, was introduced after
Freud described anxiety hysteria; we use "conversion hysteria" today as
Freud did. The third type is the obsessional neurosis, another term first
introduced by Freud that has persisted to the present.

"The opposition between the actual neuroses and the psychoneuroses
is essentially aetiological and pathogenic: the cause is definitely sexual in
both these types of neurosis, but in the former case it must be sought in 'a
disorder of [the subject's] contemporary sexual life' and not in 'important
events in his past life.' The adjective 'actual' is therefore to be understood first and foremost in the sense of *temporal* 'actuality.' In addition,
this aetiology is somatic rather than psychical: '. . . the source of excitation, the precipitating cause of the disturbance, lies in the somatic field
instead of the psychical one'" (4, p. 10).

Freud and his colleagues (especially Abraham) also created a diagnostic
system based on libidinal stages. No more than a museum piece now,

it marked a high point in the attempt to link vicissitudes of psychic development with specific disorders, embodying a theory that adult psychopathology was in direct relationship to failures to proceed along the described path of the maturbation of sexual (libidinal) life. It went like this:

The first year or so of life is lived under the domination of the oral— the most primitive—phase, in which the mouth is the principal eroto-genic zone. During the first six months of life, sucking is the infant's main activity; the baby is immersed in narcissistic gratifications that preclude awareness of a clear-cut external object. This preverbal autism is the bedrock of *schizophrenia*. In the second half of the oral stage, cannibalistic biting and devouring of a non-perceived object, in a state either of omnipotent control or of subjugation by one's object's omnipo-tence, leads to *mania* or *melancholia*. Next is the anal phase (age 2-3), again divided into two parts. In the earlier, expulsion of the ambivalently loved and hated object (as symbolized in feces) is the paradigm for *paranoia* and other non-schizophrenia *paranoid states;* in the later, pleas-ure in the power of fecal retention signifies another ambivalence—a capacity for compassion opposed by a sense of disgust. The resulting clinical state is the *compulsion neurosis.*

In the phallic phase (age 4-6) castration fears emerge in boys and penis envy in girls, the result of oedipal conflict made possible by the child's full recognition of parents as separate loved and feared objects. A pre-occupation with phallic genital pleasures and dangers underlies the future appearance of *hysteria.*

Finally, for the fortunate few, dissolution of the oedipus complex results in *mental health.*

Although the above constitutes a brilliant synthesis of theory to arrive at a diagnostic system, it was fatally flawed in not being founded on adequate data. Yet we have here a psychodynamic *theory* of diagnosis that is logical and tries to account for facts too often ignored. Freud's aim to make a diagnosis say something not only about the signs and symptoms but the underlying forces is the ideal toward which we must aim in diagnosis.

Flaws in the Analytic System

Diagnoses that are built up from an etiological base are doomed if these etiologies are false. For instance, we believe toady that a system founded on body humours (e.g., he is "melancholic" or "plegmatic") or the conjunction of stars and planets will fail (though not entirely, if its syndromes are demonstrable entities). Comparably, Freud's attempt to arrive at a diagnostic system was fatally flawed in not deriving from adequate data. Take, for example, Freud's diagnoses: neurasthenia and anxiety neurosis. First, he looked and felt he could make out two different syndromes, each of which had a different set of dynamics (different damming up of the libido) and different etiologies that caused the damming up.

> Excessive masturbation or nocturnal emissions comprised the first group of pathogenic, sexual abnormalities. They produce symptoms of fatigue, listlessness, flatulence, constipation, headache, and dyspepsia. Freud proposed that the term "neurasthenia" be henceforth limited to this group of patients alone. The second type of sexual noxa was any sexual activity which produced a state of sexual excitement or stimulation without an adequate outlet or discharge, as, for example, coitus interruptus, or love making without sexual gratification. Such activities resulted in states of anxiety, most typically in the form of anxiety attacks, and Freud proposed that such patients be diagnosed as anxiety neurosis (1, p. 187).

Errors of fact, or facts too much at the mercy of untestable theory will penetrate into a diagnosis, killing it. What are we to do with explanations built from fundamentals that are unobserved and unobservable, and have never been defined enough to gather agreement even among believers: libido as a substance that flows in and between organs, psychic energy, cathexis, neutralization, life instinct and death instinct, neuronal inertia? Or, to use the example just cited, time has simply failed to demonstrate that either masturbating or not masturbating causes psychiatric conditions. No one has ever demonstrated libido, much less the alleged biological process of "damming of the libido." Let us hope that we need not deal any longer with such diagnostic debris as "actual neurosis," "narcissistic neurosis," "pregenital conversions," "anxiety hysteria," or "transference neurosis" (when used as a diagnosis for nonpsychotic states).

A second flaw entered analytic thinking on diagnosis, one that has plagued those in other disciplines who are also looking for fundamentals: equating "concomitant" with "etiological for."

Despite the devilish temptation, neurochemists have begun resisting this idea; analysts sometimes forget. We do not always know that when we discover a dynamic at work, it is not necessarily a cause. For instance, male paranoid psychotics frequently (much more than females) suffer accusatory hallucinations of homosexuality. From this, Freud developed an etiological statement that "latent homosexuality" (in both sexes) was the cause of paranoid psychosis. There is too much other evidence today for anyone to take this seriously. It is not a law, not even a hypothesis; in fact it no longer even serves as a hunch. Yet the fact remains that the male paranoid patient usually does suffer from—is influenced by—unacceptable homosexual ideas. They just do not cause psychosis—not schizophrenia, paresis, delirium tremens, mania, nor psychosis after being hit on the head with a train.

For psychoanalysis, theory became more precious than observation, a risk any eager discipline runs when observations come forth too slowly. We try to close the gap of uncertainty by squeezing data, as if we could force them to extrude the truth.

II. The Role of Psychodynamics

Introduction: The Relation of Meaning to Behavior

Time will take care of these analytic diagnoses; they do not need us to reveal their failure. In fact, their collapse makes it too easy to dismiss the strengths that psychoanalysis can bring to diagnosis. Let us look at some of these now.

The factor that will not go away is that reified by the word "mind." No matter how taxonomists, statisticians, behaviorists, physiologists or philosophers struggle, they have not yet succeeded in removing our awareness that our behavior is usually purposeful, motivated, meaningful.*

Psychoanalysis makes one overriding contribution to our understanding of psychology. It tells us that meaning motivates behavior. Let us consider some possible motivations underlying a single overt act. I strike him—in self-defense, for he was going to hit me; or in a ritual of honor, in order to challenge him to a duel; or as part of my sexual excitement, since we are having a sado-masochistic homosexual affair; or because he is manipulating my mind with filthy remarks he secretly directs at me over the TV; or because his arrogance enrages me;

---

* "Behavior without meaning may be a reflex activity or other biological activity; it cannot be psychological activity" (6, p. 228).

or because the stage directions for the play in which we are acting demand it; or in terror, as he charges my foxhole during combat; or in jealous rage, because he stole my wife; or with paternal confidence, because he is my wayward son; or in athletic competition, during a boxing match; or without intent, while rushing amidst a crowd into a subway; or in the throes of temporal lobe seizure. To understand my striking him, then, you should want to know of more than brain function or conditioned reflexes. You must learn my intent, which depends on how I interpret the situation.

Most of the time, we sense our behavior as being soaked in meaning.* There is no way around it—there are great masses of human behavior produced by the impulses "I want" or "I do not want." No analyst would insist, however, that wishes and defenses are all there is to behavior. From Freud on, we have conceptualized a continuum of behavior with a range of causes from the primarily biological (e.g., psychomotor epilepsy) to primary psychological (e.g., student anxiety before an examination). (Our present arguments are concerned with "how much," not "either-or.")

We also should note that "cause" is relative; there are causes of causes, toward an infinite regress. For instance, the conscious meaning of a paranoid system for a patient may be that he is being threatened by strange, malignant forces. That meaning, with which he orders his perceptions as he walks down the street, may *cause* him to kill a stranger, but it does not *cause* his schizophrenia; rather, the meaning—the conviction of dire threat—was a result of an underlying process that we name "schizophrenia." This schizophrenia, let us say, was preceded by a biochemical defect, which resulted from a pathological "message," communicated by a faulty gene and transmitted over generations from a mutation, which was caused by a cosmic ray, which. . . . If, like Freud, one believes that the patient's hatred resulted from an unacceptable, and therefore unconscious, meaning—that the patient was homosexually attracted to the stranger—the unconscious meaning becomes the cause of both the murder and the schizophrenia. But if the schizophrenia in this case was a gene-controlled neurophysiological defect, meaning is not etiological for the disease though it precipitated—was the proximate motive for—the killing.

Our task is to determine which conditions are the effect of meaning

---

* However, we must be careful not to mistake a person's conviction about a meaning for necessarily being a cause.

(mind), which of body, especially brain, and which of both. The consensus nowadays is that meaning as ultimate etiology is less in most of the psychoses and greater in most of the chronic, habitual non-psychotic states that are more or less subsumed under the personality disorders or neuroses.

Analysis, then, will be most useful when behavior is especially the result of meaning. Critics to the contrary, a vast literature (not to say one's daily experience) shows how meaning—conscious and unconscious—determines behavior. Not only do we respond to the meanings we deduce as we realistically assess circumstances in the present, but we also bring habitual, lifelong interpretations to present situations—fixed attitudes and modes of expression called character structure. For instance, each time I greeted a patient at the start of an analytic hour, she would shrug her shoulders and smile sheepishly; another for months would knot her brows with angry pain; another presented a forced façade of cheery insouciance; another froze with eyes that looked blankly past. To each I appeared quite different. When their relationships with their parents were better understood, these ways of dealing with me changed. Yet, before that, each had no question, when I appeared, that he or she was responding to *me*, not to fantasies of me. Those same fixed attitudes—fantasies—had propelled their behavior with all men in authority from childhood on.

Ingrained behavior like this is ubiquitous and stamps one's view of the world. One person is "by nature" compulsively meticulous, another cautious, another cheerful, another sexually exhibitionistic. Each brings a bias to his interpretation of what is going on, and so, reading these meanings everywhere, responds predictably. And, with a good piece of analysis, we can understand rather well how these attitudes developed and why.

If constellations of behavior of such kinds can be discovered, and if they lead to maladaptations in the world, why exclude them from a list of syndromes of behavior? Yet that knowledge puts a stress on psychiatric diagnosis, introducing problems not present elsewhere in medicine. Whether these issues and the treatment questions that result can be contained in a medical model or not will not concern me now. I wish only to stress that if we can describe such syndromes and have means to study their dynamics and origins, we owe our awareness to psychodynamic studies.

This perspective—meaning organized as motive, when added to that of the organicist and behaviorist, gives a schema for etiology and dynamics that may help us some day build more sensible diagnoses. A caution: to legislate any of the three away for reasons of dogma is inexcusable.

This means confronting the neuroses and personality disorders. These states spoil our hope of a tidy, cooperative nosology: they fail to stay put as syndromes, the names and descriptions often changing; they do not fit the simpler "medical models"; they are a focus of polemics on social issues; and they make us wonder if they even are disorders when the person assigned to patient-hood often says he feels fine (or would if we would only let him be).

Example: Sexual Aberrations

These issues can be amplified with data and ideas from an aspect of my work on sexual aberrations. This will also show how I use the definition of diagnosis as syndrome, dynamics, and etiology.

With our sexual mores changing, the problem is whether one can defend the position that variations in sexual behavior—erotic or gender (i.e., masculine and feminine)—deserve to be called diagnoses. We are in danger of assigning a person a diagnosis in accord with a ruling on morality (social acceptability) promulgated by psychiatrists rather than by the meaning the behavior has for the sexual performer.

Take, for example, transvestism. Although both DSM-I and II list it, neither defines the condition, as if there were no problems in definition: for most psychiatrists, transvestism is the desire to put on clothes of the opposite sex.

If it can be shown that everyone who cross-dresses does it in more or less the same manner and circumstances and with the same conscious experiences (syndrome), from the same motivations (dynamics), and because of the same biological and/or psychological causes (etiology), then we have a diagnosis. Otherwise, we have only a symptom or sign (comparable to hallucination, which is an experience, not a diagnosis). But, before we even look at cross-dressers, the supposed unitary diagnosis crumbles in our hand when we study the texts. In one place, it is described as a form of erotic excitement; in another, as simply a desire to live in the role of the opposite sex; in another, as a form of homosexuality; and in another a likely symptom of schizophrenia. And among transvestites there is a movement (as with "homosexuals") to dictate "transvestism" as a non-diagnosis, just a different life style.

With the suspicion that there may be a number of kinds of cross-dressing, let us return to the clinical situation to see what we can learn about the process of creating a diagnosis. On doing so, we find that putting on clothes of the opposite sex has different meanings for our subjects. Some who do it are children, some adults; males may have different reasons from females; some do it to become sexually excited, some not; some want to be like a person of the opposite sex, some to make fun of a person of the opposite sex; some do it rarely, some as much as they can; some are only fooling around, some very intense; some do it intermittently, some habitually; some do it in the same style throughout their lives, others change the ways they do it; some have disorders of their sexual biology, other do not; for a few it is an essential part of a psychosis, most are not psychotic; some do it because of childhood traumas, others not; some do it as a game, some as a manifestation of an unchanging identity. How can we then consider cross-dressing—"transvestism"—a syndrome, much less a diagnosis? All that these clinical pictures have in common is the symptom of putting on the clothes of the opposite sex. This cursory sketch hints that one will not find the same underlying dynamics and causes for such a multitude of behaviors.

After observing cross-dressers for some time, I use the following classification (still being confirmed and modified by more data) that separates out a number of syndromes, for some of which I have consistently found both the same underlying dynamics and—less clearly—causative factors (7). For simplicity, I shall classify only males (though this could be achieved equally well with females).

1) *Fetishistic cross-dressing.* This is a form of fetishism, in which clothes of the opposite sex cause genital excitement. Other than one published case, it has been reported only in males. This fetishistic excitement is occasionally found in childhood, most often appears after puberty and in adolescence, but sometimes may first occur when a man is in his 30's or later. By far the greatest number of these men are overtly heterosexual and masculine in demeanor and choice of profession. Such a man knows he is a male and, the cross-dressing notwithstanding, he enjoys his maleness, as is evidenced by the keen sexual pleasure experienced in his genitals when he cross-dresses. His past history often reveals that he was cross-dressed in childhood, usually by a woman or girl who wanted to humiliate him, that is, to attack his sense of maleness and his masculinity.

2) *Effeminate homosexuality.* In this category are the boys and men who prefer males as their sex objects and whose habitual style of behavior is effeminacy. (Effeminacy means caricature of femininity, a subtly angry mimicry.) Although such males have a more than average interest in being like females, this wish is contaminated by anger toward them. Typically found in childhood is a mother who has mixed together an excessive intimacy and overconcern for her son with punishment and anger aimed especially at those behaviors she thinks are precursors of masculinity. An ordinarily masculine father is not reported in these cases.

3) *True transsexualism.* Although the term "transsexual" is used often nowadays to label anyone requesting sex-change, that use is too broad, covering several different conditions. I refer here to an anatomically normal male who has been feminine (not effeminate) since earliest childhood and has never had any episodes, momentary or extended, when he could function or appear as masculine. Although knowing he is a male, he says he nonetheless feels he is somehow a female and therefore would like his body changed to conform to his identity. He is exclusively erotically aroused by other males but feels he is heterosexual, using as evidence his sense of self rather than his genitals. His identification with femininity is not contaminated by hostility but is rather the result of a blissful symbiosis with mother from birth through later childhood, with the result that he does not have the opportunity to experience or appreciate masculinity. His father, though usually still a member of the household, is psychologically absent and rarely encountered by the child.

4) *"Transsexualism."* In this category, separate from the last, are males requesting sex-change but who look clinically different, have different life histories, different dynamics, and different causative factors in childhood (cf. 5). These males have not been feminine from earliest childhood on and are not feminine now; rather they strongly express qualities like those of effeminate homosexuals or fetishistic cross-dressers. In none are the same dynamics and the same family etiological factors found as in the feminine, true transsexuals.

5) *Intersexuality.* These are the people with one or another of the biological disorders of maleness and femaleness, in which a fetal patho-neurophysiology (often genetic) causes aberrant masculinity or femininity, with associated cross-dressing.

6) *Hermaphroditic identity.* These people, because of ambiguous genitals at birth, are not clearly assigned to one sex or the other. Because

the family incessantly communicates—grossly or subliminally—to the child that it is not a normal person but rather is in some way of equivocal sex, the child grows up with a disturbance in masculinity or femininity that precisely matches the family's communications about the child's sex. This condition should be distinguished from the previous one, in which the intersexuality itself is the driving force behind the changed gender identity (as in some patients with Klinefelter's—XXY—syndrome). In the present situation, it is not an innate, biological "force" that causes the cross-gender impulses, but rather the family's attitudes from infancy on.

7) *Psychosis.* In psychoses, especially among males, one frequently finds hallucinations and delusions relating to the patient's uncertainties about the intactness of his gender identity. Much less frequently, psychotic patients will act on the impulses underlying the symptoms and will behave in some manner related to behavior of the opposite sex. This may include cross-dressing. At times, the cross-dressing produces a rather natural approximation to that of the opposite sex, but often it is, rather, a bizarre display, fully infiltrated with the psychotic thinking.

8) *Casual cross-dressing.* Most of the boys who cross-dress are merely experimenting when putting on clothes of the opposite sex. The activity fails to stir them, and so there are not the long-term effects seen in the above categories. Likewise, men, especially in carnival situations, may cross-dress for the moment, the essential reason being a show and a display of humor that is meant to make fun mildly of women. Although an analyst might find dynamics at work related to identification with women, the depth and intensity of these are too slight to be equivalent to those found in the above categories.

Recognizing that one can find cases less pure than those cited,* I still believe the above is a usable classification, containing within it the means —syndrome, dynamics, and etiology—for accurate diagnostic work. If this is possible with gender identity and its disorders, cannot something like it be done for other kinds of the habitual behavior patterns that we call personality disorders? And, if we make it clear that we are not using diagnoses as a surreptitious means of insulting others, or worse, of reducing their civil rights, we may still talk of these constellations as disorders or conditions or states without the diagnoses indicating an intent to moralize. Only when a sense of badness is in the dynamics—

---

* For which we can perhaps use the pseudo-diagnosis "Mixed Group."

actually experienced by the aberrant person—should it be connoted in the diagnosis. I shall discuss this now in regard to the term "perversion."

Sexual Aberrations: Variants of Perversions

There is strong evidence that the just-noted sense of being bad results from desires to harm one's sex objects (8). So, in line with my way of defining "diagnosis," let me circle back on the category "sexual deviations" once more, drawing on my research to show how a psychodynamic viewpoint sorts out diagnostic issues. In no other category are we more likely to run into confusion introduced by social concerns.* Trying to bring objectivity to perceptions of sexual perceptions of sexual behavior, our psychiatric forebears tried to launder their disgust of "perversion." They brought forth a progression of terms (within which were contained, among others, sexual deviants) from "constitutional psychopathic inferior," to "psychopathic personality," to "sociopathic personality" to arrive at "sexual deviation"; even this last will now be changed. They wished not to be pejorative, but, as usual, changing words in the diagnoses did not change attitudes.

Despite hard thought, we do not yet use consistent criteria for calling a sexual act aberrant. The words "aberrant," "deviant," or "variant" have a statistical implication, connoting that a minority of a population indulges in the behavior. That is too vague; and, when we seek out those to whom we shall ascribe normal behavior, we find they are so rare that they are statistically as deviant as the rest. Some equate "heterosexuality" with normality, but there is certainly enough aberrance in "heterosexuality" to make it meaningless as a baseline.

Other criteria have been used to define aberrance: the sex or species of one's object; is the object living, dead, or inanimate by nature; orifices used; society's attitudes (such as religious injunctions, laws, peer group pressures), and more. But these are subject to moralistic judgments, too easily contaminated by the diagnoser's opinions of what does or does not represent Natural Law. None of that should be the business of diagnosis.

It seems to me, that we are more consistent if, in identifying behavior as sexually aberrant, we determine the meaning of the act for the aberrant person, even if this is more easily described in theory than put into practice. Using that approach, I suggest the following diagnostic outline.

---

* The same issue of immorality once joined "sexual deviations" to "sociopathic personality" (DSM-I).

The genetic term is "aberrations," to be divided into two subcategories —"variant" and "perversion"—distinguished from each other by differences in clinical picture (syndrome), dynamics, and etiology.

By *aberration* I mean an erotic technique or constellation of techniques that one uses as his complete sexual act and that differs from his culture's traditional, avowed definition of normality.

By *variant* (or deviation) I mean an aberration that is not primarily the staging of forbidden fantasies, especially fantasies of harming others. Examples would be behavior set off only by abnormal brain activity, as with a tumor, experimental drug, or electrical impulse from an implanted electrode; or an aberrant act one is driven to *faute de mieux;* or sexual experiments one does from curiosity and finds not exciting enough to repeat.

Perversion, the erotic form of hatred, is a fantasy, usually acted out but occasionally restricted to a daydream (either self-produced or packaged by others, that is, pornography). It is a habitual, preferred aberration necessary for one's full satisfaction, primarily motivated by hostility. By "hostility" I mean a state in which one wishes to harm an object; that differentiates it from "aggression," which often implies only forcefulness. The hostility in perversion takes form in a fantasy of revenge hidden in the actions that make up the perversion and serves to convert childhood trauma to adult triumph. To create the greatest excitement, the perversion must also portray itself as an act of risk-taking.

While these definitions remove former incongruities, they impose on us the new burden of learning from a person what motivates him. But we are freed from a process of designation that did not take the subject's personality and motivation into account. We no longer need to define a perversion according to the anatomy used, the object chosen, the society's stated morality, or the number of people who do it. All we need know is what it means to the person doing it; while this may be difficult for us to uncover, there is still no a priori reason to reject this technique for defining. (These definitions are taken from and discussed at greater length in [8].)

Before rejecting this dissection of sexual aberrations, one can recall that we followed the same logic when distinguishing, in DSM-I, between "antisocial reaction" and "dyssocial reaction," or the permutation taken by this sensible idea in DSM-II, wherein "antisocial personality" is distinguished from "dyssocial behavior," the latter—comparable to my use of "variant"—now recognized as one of the "conditions without manifest psychiatric disorder and nonspecific conditions."

CONCLUSIONS

It has become stylish in some circles to dismiss psychodynamics from diagnostic considerations. To do so requires an act of faith, a belief that one's behavior is not motivated by the meanings one reads into the world. Although any of us can show that the diagnoses of psychoanalysis did not work, we can show only that they failed because their data were flawed. So let us be cautious, keeping alive the idea that a proper diagnosis should signify the forces that create behavior. That implies the mind, that mass of thoughts, feelings, memories, fantasies, perceptions, attitudes, desires, and defenses organized so as to give a continuity of meaning to one's life.

Inventors of diagnostic systems who ignore this will not extricate psychiatry from its diagnostic dilemmas.

REFERENCES

1. Brenner, C. *An Elementary Textbook of Psychoanalysis* (2nd edition). New York: Doubleday, 1974.
2. Fleiss, R. *The Psychoanalytic Reader*, Vol. I. New York: International Universities Press, 1948.
3. Goldman, R. *Principles of Medical Science*. New York: McGraw-Hill Book Company, 1973.
4. LaPlanche, J. & Pontalis, J.-B. *The Language of Psycho-Analysis*. London: Hogarth Press, 1973.
5. Person, E. S., & Oversey, L. The transsexual syndrome in males, I and II, *Amer. J. Psychotherapy*, 28:4-20-174-193, 1974.
6. Schafer, R. *A New Language for Psychoanalysis*. New Haven: Yale University Press, 1976.
7. Stoller, R. J. The term "transvestism." *Arch. Gen. Psychiat.*, 24:230-237, 1971.
8. Stoller, R. J. *Perversion*. New York: Pantheon, 1975.

3

Neuropsychological Concepts and Psychiatric Diagnosis

RALPH M. REITAN, PH.D.

The theme of this Symposium, oriented toward new evidence as a basis for reconsideration of existing categories of psychiatric diagnosis, clearly points toward the biological bases for behavioral disorders. Such an orientation could have considerable significance in the area of psychiatry with respect to changing emphases and even directions of clinical practice.

Psychiatry has tended in many respects to ignore biological bases of behavior in terms of genetic influences as well as conditions that may lead to subtle deterioration of brain functions. Psychiatry has been moving farther and farther away during the past several decades from the fields represented by the neurological sciences. This trend very possibly has been quite understandable in consideration of limited conceptual and practical progress toward elucidation of the biological bases of mental disorders. However, during the past two to three decades there has been some substantial progress made in the study of human brain-behavior relationships. This latter development has tended to pursue its own course largely separate from the course of clinical psychiatry. It appears at present that the time may well have come for a more intensive consideration of the complementary aspects of developments in the area of brain-behavior relationships with respect to psychiatric diagnosis and treatment. For example, we have recently learned much about the differential functions of the two cerebral hemispheres, specialization of abilities within the brain, and even of intra-hemispheric behavioral characteristics. Further, the differential psychological correlates of various types of brain involvement have been demonstrated. The reversibility of deficits associated with brain lesions, which have been assumed in many instances to be non-reversible, have been documented. The interaction of biological and environmental influences has been clearly demonstrated. We have come to realize that the brain is the organ of behavior, that everyone's brain is trained by environmental experiences, and that significant training and influence on eventual behavior are possible even in persons with damaged or impaired brains.

Although there has been a strong contingent of biologically oriented psychiatrists who have made significant contributions to understanding of brain-behavior relationships, the time appears to have arrived for additional disciplines to make their contribution to the understanding of disordered behavior as well. Clinical neuropsychology is a relatively new field, and its entire orientation has been directed toward understanding of brain-behavior relationships. Thus, a biologically oriented approach toward elucidation of behavioral deviations is entirely consistent with the entire history of clinical neuropsychology and the concepts and results developed in this field may now be of significance for clinical psychiatric application.

Standards of Evidence that Are Needed

Geschwind (10) has recently presented a rather typical overview of the areas of neurology and psychiatry, noting the fact that many persons who are observed initially to have emotional or psychiatric problems eventually are determined to have some type of brain lesion or brain dysfunction. He emphasizes the need for careful neurological examination and diagnosis in psychiatric patients, although recognizing that many behavioral disturbances will not be found to have an organic basis. He notes that psychiatric disorders may be diagnosed as organic disease and that irreversible organic disease may be diagnosed as a functional disorder. He goes on to cite instances in which behavioral disorders were initially prominent and psychiatric diagnoses established, but in which the patients were later found to have lesions such as a glioblastoma multiforme, a craniopharyngioma, a subfrontal tumor, and Huntington's chorea. Geschwind's presumption is that the neurological disorder was responsible for the behavioral disturbance.

While this may certainly have been true, the conclusion would be convincingly established only if we knew the necessary and sufficient conditions whereby such lesions would give rise to the behavioral deviations that were observed. Not knowing these conditions, the biological bases for the behavioral disturbances are rendered rather presumptive and, in fact, citation of such instances has probably actually tended to undercut the significance of neurological deficits (because of their rareness, if nothing else) as a basis for behavioral change. Such lesions are *not* found in most persons with psychiatric disorders. However, neurological changes of a more subtle nature than customarily revealed by clinical neurological examinations may be of definite significance in causing behavioral disturbances of a psychiatric nature. The critical point is that we not only be able to identify individual persons who have behavioral disturbances followed by diagnosis of a brain lesion but that we have learned enough about brain-behavior relationships, throughout the full range of individuals involved, to be able to identify biological deviations, specifically for the individual patients, on the basis of unique behavioral changes. Only through meeting such requirements will our knowledge be sufficiently detailed and secure to permit application in the area of psychiatric diagnosis and practice.

A Brief Review of Biological Factors in Major Mental Disorder

Deviations of biological functioning in psychiatric conditions have been demonstrated for many years and continue to be documented further. Mirsky (32) reviewed some of these findings, especially dealing with EEG studies in schizophrenic and comparison samples, and concluded that schizophrenics show certain abnormalities that are not seen in normal subjects. He also briefly reviewed several additional papers pointing toward the presence of positive neuropathological findings in schizophrenic patients, although the question still exists as to whether these morphological changes may be related only incidentally to the psychiatric state.

Difficult problems exist in this area because of possible differing criteria with respect to the diagnosis of schizophrenia. However, Haug (13) reported pneumoencephalographic and clinical findings in a series of 278 mental patients. He focused particularly on schizophrenic patients and found that 61% of 137 patients showed an abnormal pneumoencephalogram. The mean size of various parts of the ventricular system was larger in the schizophrenic than in the group with non-organic mental disorders, although the largest mean ventricular sizes were recorded in a group with organic mental disorders. While about two-thirds of the schizophrenic patients had abnormal pneumoencephalograms, Haug also analyzed the data in more detail. Among the 137 schizophrenic patients, he omitted 36 because he was able to identify various complicating disorders such as head trauma, alcoholism, prior leukotomy, or advanced age. Among the remaining 101 schizophrenics, all below the age of 60 years and representing various types of schizophrenia, he found abnormal pneumoencephalograms in 58%. Although no differences were present among hebephrenic, catatonic, and paranoid schizophrenics, some evidence was present to indicate that the degree of mental deterioration correlated with the degree of ventricular enlargement. Of 46 highly impaired schizophrenics, only 9 (20%) had normal pneumoencephalograms. While findings of this kind do not necessarily imply a direct causal relationship (many patients with ventricular enlargement or even definite cerebral atrophy show no evidence of schizophrenia), they do definitely point toward biological changes of the brain in schizophrenics as compared with control groups. It is interesting to note that over the years neuropsychological examination of many patients with ventricular enlargement and cerebral atrophy (although without psychosis) consistently has shown evidence of serious neuropsychological impairment on measures that will be discussed below.

Shagass (41) has presented an extensive and detailed review of electroencephalography and evoked potentials in psychotic patients. He has compared particularly the major findings in affective psychoses with those in schizophrenia. Shagass identifies many electroencephalographic and evoked response measures which show differences between mentally ill persons and normals, as well as between schizophrenic patients and patients with affective psychoses. However, he points out that psychiatric electrophysiology is still at an early state of development and it is difficult at this point to relate particular EEG or evoked response characteristics to specific diagnostic categories.

The work of Meltzer and his associates, concerned with skeletal muscle and subterminal motorneuron abnormalities in patients with schizophrenia and affective psychoses, has produced some exciting and provocative findings. The majority of such patients appeared to demonstrate abnormalities, including: 1) increased activity in serum of skeletal-muscle type creatine phosphokinase (CPK) and aldolase activity (20-23,

27, 28, 30, 31); 2) abnormal extrafusal muscle fibers in skeletal muscle biopsies (5, 22, 29); and 3) abnormalities of subterminal motorneurons (25, 26). Meltzer reports that he observed no differences among groups of psychotic patients in increased CPK activity, having studied groups with acute and chronic schizophrenia, unipolar and bipolar affective psychoses, non-psychotic psychiatric patients, and normal controls; but in 25% of the psychotic patients the peak increase was equal to or greater than five times the upper limit of normal. Rowland (38) has pointed out that increased CPK levels occur in many neuromuscular as well as nervous system disorders and the significance of increased serum CPK in acute psychoses at this point represents an unanswered question. However, the possibility exists that these serum enzyme changes reflect some neuropathic or myopathic disorder directly related to cerebral abnormality which, in turn, may be related to psychotic behavior.

Slater and his associates (42, 43) have emphasized the significance of biological disorders related to brain functions in other groups of persons with emotional disorders. Slater and Glithero (43) did follow-ups on 99 patients who, seven to eleven years earlier, had been diagnosed as having hysterical reactions. They were able to obtain follow-up information on 85 of these patients. Eight of them had died of various organic illnesses which the authors feel were probably present at the time of the initial diagnosis of hysteria, 19 had received diagnoses of organic illnesses together with the original diagnosis of hysteria, 22 had developed organic illnesses that probably were present but undetected when the diagnosis of hysteria was originally made, and 32 patients showed no evidence of organic disease. The authors conclude that unrecognized and undiagnosed organic disease may well be a significant factor among patients who are initially diagnosed as showing evidence of hysteria. The authors also postulate that organic disease may bring about a general disturbance of personality adjustment which may in turn cause affective lability, hypochondriasis, attention-seeking, self-concern, suggestibility, and variability of symptoms.

These citations serve only as examples that somatic disorders may, in many instances, be of significance with respect to psychiatric diagnoses. They do not, however, provide any convincing information to the effect that we have a fundamental grasp of the specific biological disorders that may represent necessary and sufficient conditions to produce psychopathology.

Interaction of Neurological and Psychiatric Deficits and
Approaches Toward Neuropsychological Measurements

Lipowski (17) believes that the neglect of cerebral disease or disorder in producing pathology has resulted partly from the tendencies among some biologically oriented scientists to attempt to explain all mental illness in terms of demonstrated neuropathology. Obviously, the fact that a patient may have a brain lesion and previously have manifested a psychiatric disorder is scarcely a compelling explanation of the role of the brain lesion in the person's mental illness. Thus, this approach has been rather restricted in terms of its explanatory contribution. However, a tendency to ignore cerebral changes has led to a complete disregard of somatic factors as having some type of etiologic role in psychiatric disorders. An equally restricted focus, as pointed out by Lipowski, has resulted from purely psychological explanatory hypotheses as the chief orientation in understanding psychopathology.

Lipowski believes that there are three major classes of psychiatric disorders that are causally related to organic disease. These include: 1) organic brain syndromes resulting from brain damage or temporary metabolic derangement of brain functions; 2) reactive syndromes represented by maladaptive modes of coping with somatic or cerebral disease and the distressing psychological and social consequences; and 3) deviant behavior directly stemming from the presence of illness such as lack of compliance or avoidance of medical management, massive denial of illness, regressive dependence, and other forms of maladaptive responses.

Lipowski has cited the possibly antiquated nature and ambiguous meaning of the term "dementia," although many neurologists think of dementia as representing a major area of overlap with psychiatric disorder and neurological deficit. Generally, the term dementia has been thought to refer to a rather global impairment of cognitive and intellectual functions that is fairly severe in nature and represents progressive deterioration. In this sense, the term is not particularly meaningful inasmuch as the classification neglects persons with relatively lesser degrees of impairment. Lipowski points out that dementia, like any other syndrome, has degrees of severity and may be present in mild forms as well as in more severe forms. In fact, while dementia is customarily viewed as involving rather general intellectual and cognitive deterioration as well as memory impairment, other evidence suggests that the essential feature may relate to abstraction and organizing ability. Basically, dementia is a term that refers clinically to deterioration of efficiency in performance rather than to loss of any specific and highly defined adaptive skills. In fact, loss of abstraction, reasoning ability, and ability to understand the essential nature of problems represents just the kind of fundamental deficit implied by the term "dementia" and also represents the most common manifestation of impaired brain functions that has yet been measured (33).

Thus, the role of impairment in abstraction ability and efficiency of intellectual and cognitive performance, very commonly manifested in persons with brain lesions, must undoubtedly be a major factor in the occurrence of confusional states, anxiety, and overall inadequacy of adjustment. In fact, we postulate that the frequent references to alteration of the individual's characteristic personality style and behavioral traits, often referred to as personality change, is intimately related to abstraction and reasoning ability. Halstead observed changes of this kind in association with brain lesions many years ago (12) and developed a specific test for this kind of ability which has been found to reflect the effects of impairment of brain functions more consistently than any other test reported in the literature (33, 37). In an operational approach regarding the complementary aspects of clinical neuropsychology and psychiatric diagnosis, a careful examination of the nature of this test is of importance.

Wechsler devised measures of intellectual function for normal subjects. Ward Halstead, in 1935, began the first full-time laboratory for study of higher-level psychological functions of patients with brain lesions. Halstead's approach was to engage initially in a naturalistic kind of experiment. He observed patients with brain lesions while in their homes, at work, in recreational settings, and in as many real-life situations as he could. In this way he was able to formulate hypotheses regarding the specific kinds of deficits that persons with brain lesions demonstrated. On the basis of these observations he returned to his laboratory and attempted to devise standardized experiments which could be applied to measure such deficits. He developed a battery of tests which have been shown (34) to be much more sensitive to cerebral damage than are the Wechsler Scales and also, curiously, to have much less of an intercorrelation among themselves than do the Wechsler subtests. This latter finding suggests that Halstead's Tests cover much more ground with respect to the range of their measurement.

While Halstead's complete battery cannot be demonstrated in this paper, it has recently been described in full detail (37). It is important, nevertheless, in the present context to present some notion of the types of intellectual and, when intact, cognitive functions that seem particularly susceptible to brain damage and representative of normal brain functioning. One of the most useful and valid tests developed by Halstead was his Category Test. This procedure utilizes an apparatus for successive projection of 208 stimulus figures on a screen in front of the patient. The testing procedure, which is actually a standardized experiment, proceeds as follows. After viewing each stimulus-figure, the patient selects an answer by depressing any one of four levers labeled 1, 2, 3, and 4. A harsh buzzer sounds if the "wrong" lever is depressed, whereas a pleasant bell sounds if the answer is correct. Before the test begins, the subject is informed that the test is divided into several groups of items and that in each group a single principle underlies the correct response for each item. On the first item in a group the subject can only guess at the right answer, but, as he progresses through the items, the bell or

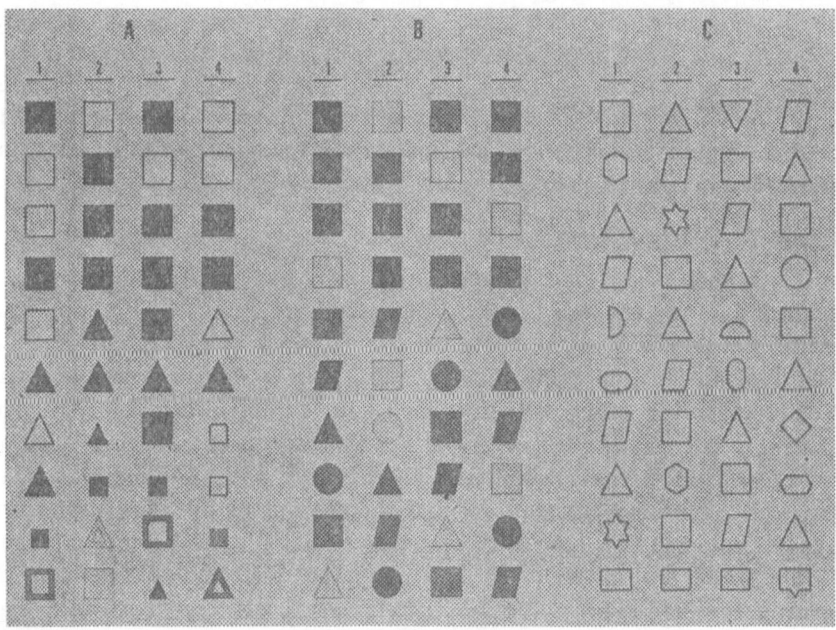

Figure 1. Illustration of the content included in the Halstead Category Test for measuring abstraction abilities dependent on brain functions.

buzzer accompanying each response permits testing of one possible principle after another until the solution is found.

Since the Category Test illustrates the kinds of mental processes that are among the most vulnerable to the impairing effects of cerebral damage, an illustration (not based on the actual principles used in the test) is presented in Figure 1.

Begin with Column A. Remember that a single principle governs the "correct" answer for each item in the column. Answers should be given by selection of items 1, 2, 3, or 4 for each figure. It is possible to derive information from "wrong" as well as "right" answers, since a wrong answer provides evidence for eliminating irrelevant or incorrect principles. A correct answer is more helpful in a positive way, however, because it may offer substantiation of the correct principle. Beware of the possibility of correct answers given for the wrong reason, since these can be very costly in one's attempt to solve the problem.

Expose the correct answers for the first column, given at the end of this sentence, one at a time and only after having first responded to each item: 2, 1, 3, 4, 2, 4, 2, 3, 2, 2. Even though you may have answered more than a "chance" number correct, the principle may not be entirely clear to you. This frequently happens with persons with normal brain functions and, in its own right, serves to illustrate the relatively loose coupling that frequently exists between rational behavior and one's ability to explain verbally why the behavior was rational. The principle governing correct choices in the first column is quite simple—the correct answer for each item was the number of solid as contrasted with outlined figures.

The types of reasoning, abstraction, or concept-formation processes needed for this test are further illustrated in Column B, but now the principle governing correct choices has changed. The answers for the ten items in Column B are 2, 3, 4, 1, 3, 2, 2, 4, 3, 1. The principle again was simple, even though the diversity of the stimulus material may have confused the issue. One of the basic characteristics of this test is to identify those persons who can recognize and then ignore extraneous aspects of the stimulus material and thereby get to the essential nature of the problem. This type of intelligence is related to, but rather different from, formal educational training or IQ, and differentiates persons with normal and damaged brains. The principle was to select the answer corresponding to the position of the lightest figure in each item.

Column C presents a more difficult set of items. Again, one can only guess on the first item. This is unimportant because the test results are principally a function of how much one can learn from his mistakes as well as his successes. The answers for the third column are as follows: 3, 1, 2, 4, 1, 3, 4, 2, 1, 4. The principle was to select the number of the figure in each item that did not have a horizontal base. The Halstead Category Test requires the use of mental processes that are fundamental to practical intelligence. The subject must observe similarities and differences of the stimulus material, both within single items and between successive items. In other words, the first requirement is for careful observation and discerning description of the elements of the problem. Next, the subject must postulate a reasonable principle for organization of the similarities and differences in the stimulus material. He must be ready to reject or modify this principle according to new facts as they appear in successive items. Finally, he must face up to the consequences of his decisions as represented by the bell and buzzer for right and wrong answers. If his answers are wrong, he must have the adaptability, flexibility, and patience to go on searching for the correct answer.

Technically, this test is described as measuring abstraction, concept-formation, and organizational ability. When one considers the nature of the task, it is not surprising that the results on the Category Test are highly effective in showing the significant but subtle and sometimes elusive kinds of deficits that are frequently present in persons with cerebral lesions. Interestingly, the ability to perform well on this test also drops off with advancing age more rapidly than does performance on most psychological tests (36).

CASE W.P.:

An Illustration of Neuropsychological Data Sufficient to Require a Conclusion of Cerebral Pathology

Examination of this patient's brain after his death made it quite clear that he had a significant lesion of the left temporal lobe in addition to the more obvious lesion of the right cerebral hemisphere. Although clinical evaluation before surgery had suggested the presence of dysphasia, the clinical diagnosis emphasized only the involvement of the right cerebral hemisphere. In neuropsychological evaluation, however, we have focused on the necessary and sufficient evidence for brain lesions and the data from neuropsychological testing forced us to conclude that bilateral damage was present. The fact that the data derived from neuropsychological examination may *require* a conclusion of cerebral damage, even in the individual subject, is of potential importance in differentiating among psychiatric patients those deficits which are only incidentally related to biological determinants as contrasted with those deficits which require a conclusion of biological disorder.

This 61-year-old man had completed high school and had gone to college for a period of time but was not able to remember just how much college work he had completed. For about one year he had experienced difficulty in walking and had become quite forgetful, being unable to remember the names even of close friends. About three months prior to admission to our Medical Center he suffered a seizure that consisted of turning of the head and eyes to the right. He was then admitted to a local hospital where studies, including an angiogram, suggested the possibility of a tumor in the right cerebral hemisphere. The patient was admitted to our hospital for further and repeated evaluation. Physical neurological examination showed evidence of weakness of the left upper eyelid and some droop of the corner of the mouth on the left side. It was difficult to perform a sensory examination reliably because the patient was not able to respond very well. He himself seemed to recognize that his intellectual functions had declined. He gave his age incorrectly as 58 and demonstrated other evidence of disorientation with respect to time. The examination suggested that the patient had some dysstereognosis on the left, although he also seemed to have some weakness and dyspraxia of his left upper extremity. He was also impaired in his ability to walk. However, the patient did demonstrate some dressing dyspraxia and it appeared that dysphasia also was present.

Bilateral cerebral angiograms were performed which showed a definite shift of the paracallosal vessels to the left under the falx, with elevation of the right Sylvian vessels. A large area of tumor stain was visible in the medial and lateral aspects of the anterior portion of the right temporal lobe. EEG showed evidence of Delta waves, Grade II, in the right Sylvian area. Neuropsychological examination was performed 11 days after admission and the patient was operated 21 days after admission. Partial removal of a tumor in the right temporal area was perfromed. It appeared at the time of surgery that there was extensive infiltration of the tumor in the right temporal lobe and probably posteriorly in the right cerebral hemisphere. Although the patient showed some mild improvement following the operation, his general physical condition began

TABLE 1

Results of Neuropsychological Examination

PATIENT: ......; AGE: *61*; SEX: *M*; EDUCATION: *12*; HANDEDNESS: *R*

WECHSLER-BELLEVUE SCALE (FORM I)

VIQ	79
PIQ	84
FS IQ	74
VWS	16
PWS	4
Total WS	20
Information	7
Comprehension	6
Digit Span	0
Arithmetic	0
Similarities	3
Vocabulary	8
Picture Arrangement	1
Picture Completion	2
Block Design	1
Object Assembly	0
Digit Symbol	0

TRAIL MAKING TEST *

Part A: ___ seconds, ___ errors
Part B: ___ seconds, ___ errors

* CANNOT PERFORM

STRENGTH OF GRIP

Dominant hand: 26.5 kilograms
Non-dominant hand: 16.5 kilograms

MILES ABC TEST
OF OCULAR DOMINANCE

Right: 9 Left: 1

REITAN-KLOVE
TACTILE FORM RECOGNITION TEST

Dominant hand: 0 errors, ___ seconds
Non-dominant hand: 4 errors, ___ seconds

HALSTEAD'S NEUROPSYCHOLOGICAL TEST BATTERY

Category Test _____ 157

Tactual Performance Test
Dominant hand: 15.0 (2 IN)
Non-dominant hand: 15.0 (0 IN)
Both hands: 15.0 (2 IN)

Total Time 45.0
Memory 1
Localization 1

Seashore Rhythm Test
Raw Score: 13 _____ 10

Speech-sounds Perception Test _____ 26

Finger Oscillation Test _____ 45
Dominant hand: 45
Non-dominant hand: 37

IMPAIRMENT INDEX: 1.0

REITAN-INDIANA APHASIA SCREENING TEST

PATIENT: _____

Copy SQUARE	Repeat TRIANGLE "Tri................angle"
Name SQUARE	Repeat MASSACHUSETTS "Mashashooshess"
Spell SQUARE "C-q-u-a-r-e". Patient knew "c" was wrong but couldn't correct it.	Repeat METHODIST EPISCOPAL "Methodist Epistical"
Copy CROSS	Write SQUARE
Name CROSS	Read SEVEN Patient counted on fingers, but OK.
Spell CROSS "S-r-o-c - S-r-o-s-s - c-r-o;s-c-r-o-s-s"	Repeat SEVEN
Copy TRIANGLE	Repeat/Explain HE SHOUTED THE WARNING. Repeated "morning" instead of warning. Explained:"Helping?
Name TRIANGLE "T-r-i-a-n-q-l-e....no"	Write HE SHOUTED THE WARNING. I'd be asking for help, wouldn't I?"
Spell TRIANGLE	Compute 85 - 27 = Examiner questioned patient about (-). "Oh no"; wanted to do it again.
Name BABY	Compute 17 X 3 = Examiner gave 8 X 3. "21"
Write CLOCK	Name KEY "A lock locker."
Name FORK	Demonstrate use of KEY
Read 7 SIX 2 "7". Patient told to read it all. OK.	Draw KEY
Read MGW "GWM"	Read PLACE LEFT HAND TO RIGHT EAR. "That's my right." Upon repeated promptings, OK.
Reading I "See the black fog - dog"	Place LEFT HAND TO RIGHT EAR Placed right hand to right ear, self-corrected.
Reading II "He is a fiendly animal a famous winter-wonder-of dog shows. Wonder..wonder."	Place LEFT HAND TO LEFT ELBOW "I don't have any." On questioning he tried and shook his head.

REITAN-KLOVE SENSORY-PERCEPTUAL EXAMINATION

(Instance indicated where stimulus was not perceived or was incorrectly perceived.)

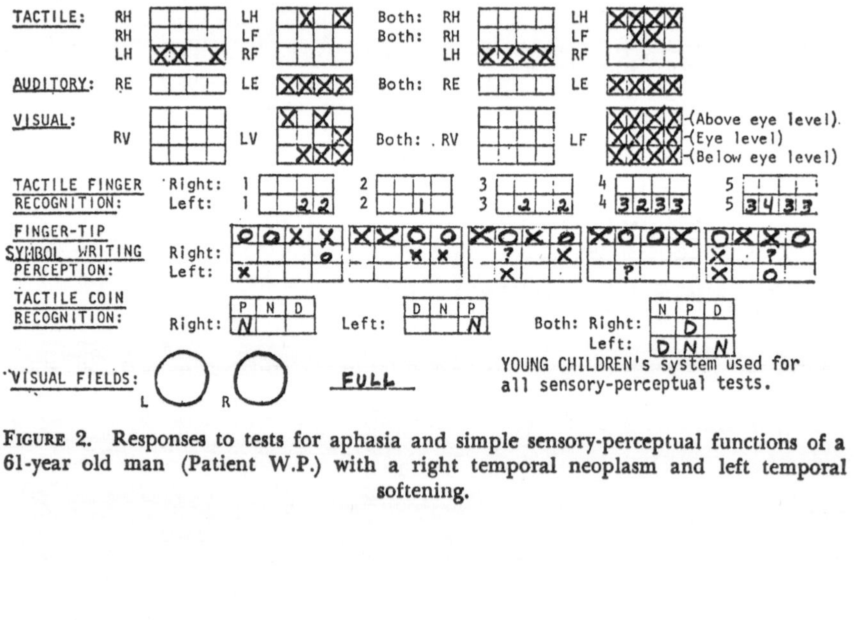

FIGURE 2. Responses to tests for aphasia and simple sensory-perceptual functions of a 61-year old man (Patient W.P.) with a right temporal neoplasm and left temporal softening.

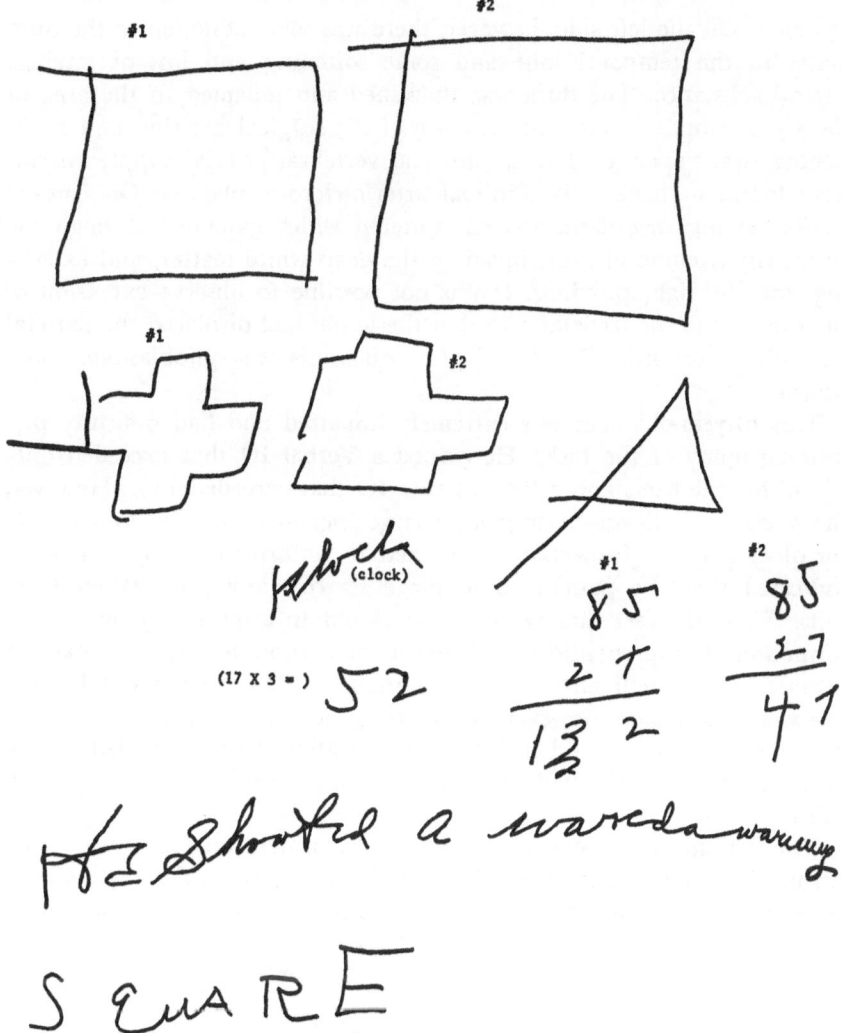

FIGURE 3. Simple drawing, writing, and calculating efforts of Patient W. P.

to deteriorate about 2 months later and continued to the point of his death about 71 days after surgery was performed.

Autopsy revealed that both cerebral hemispheres showed a great amount of swelling with enlargement of the gyri and diminution of the sulci. The right cerebral hemisphere was shifted to the left and the right lateral ventricle had crossed the midline, impinging on the left lateral ventricle. On the left side, however, there was some adhesion to the dura mater in the temporal lobe and some softening and loss of cerebral cirtical substance. The dura was thickened and inflamed in the area of the right temporal lobe and evidence of the surgical excision and tissue removal was apparent. The carotid and vertebral arterial supply systems were found to have only minimal arteriosclerotic plagues. On coronal section, a huge neoplasm was encountered which extended through the entire right temporal area, invading the deep white matter, and extending into the right pulvinar. It was not possible to observe extension of the tumor into the parietal area, but the lesion had displaced the parietal operculum upward. The histological diagnosis was glioblastoma multiforme.

This 61-year-old man was extremely impaired and had difficulty performing many of the tasks. He earned a Verbal IQ that exceeded only 8% of his age peers and a Performance IQ that exceeded 14%. However, the Wechsler-Bellevue Scale gives a large increment in Performance IQ for older persons. Inspection of the actual Performance weighted scores indicated that the patient could make scarcely any progress on these tests. Thus, the fact that he was able to obtain some credit on the Information, Comprehension, and Vocabulary subtests suggests that his actual Verbal intelligence was higher than his Performance intelligence. We would postulate, however, considering the patient's previous employment as an engineer and his years of education, that his verbal intelligence has been strikingly depressed although he still has some abilities in this regard.

The patient also demonstrated severe impairment on Halstead's Tests, earning an Impairment Index of 1.0 (Table 1). He was able to make little progress on the Category Test, was so confused that he was not able to

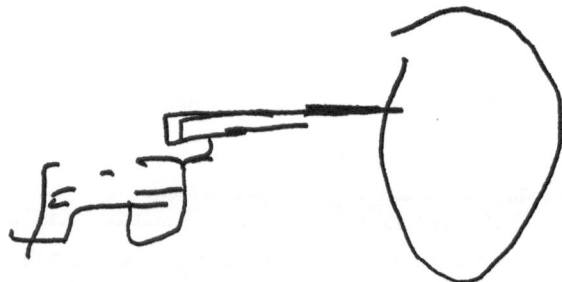

FIGURE 4. Attempt of Patient W. P. to copy a key.

perform the Trail Making Test at all, and remembered only one of the shapes after a 45-minute blindfolded exposure to the Tactual Performance Test. Finger-tapping speed was not markedly reduced in the right (preferred) upper extremity for a person of this age, but his finger-tapping speed was a little slow with the left hand as compared with the right hand. Although the patient was grossly impaired on the Tactual Performance Test in general, it appeared that he was able to make a little progress when using only the right and when using both hands. However, he was unable to make any progress with his left hand. Thus, the results at this point suggested that the patient may have a little impairment on the left side of his body and that his Performance IQ may be somewhat more impaired than his Verbal IQ. In addition, however, the results quite clearly indicate that the patient was grossly and severely impaired on tests sensitive to the condition of his brain and that his brain was seriously and severely compromised biologically.

Additional results should be noted. For example, the patient's grip strength was clearly more reduced on the left side than the right. He had a number of sensory-perceptual deficits that were more prominent on the left side (Figure 2). For example, in tactile form recognition he made no errors with his right hand but four errors in 8 trials with his left hand. He also demonstrated pronounced sensory losses on the left side. The patient apparently had some left hypesthesia, judging from the fact that he failed occasionally to report unilateral stimuli on the left side. With bilateral simultaneous stimulation, however, the patient rather consistently failed to report the stimulus given to his left hand and occasionally failed to report the stimulus to his left face when it was in competition with a stimulus to the right hand. We were not able to elicit even unilateral responses to auditory stimulation on the left side and the patient also showed a definite tendency to fail to perceive unilateral visual stimulation on the left side. Judging from the procedure used in our examination, it is somewhat difficult to note if he had a primary auditory or visual loss on the left side as contrasted with a tendency, seen in some patients, to be able to respond on the affected side only with a complete absence of surrounding or competing stimuli. In tests for tactile finger localization the patient had no difficulty whatsoever on his right hand but made many mistakes on his left hand. This finding would tend to suggest that the parietal area of the left cerebral hemisphere was in better biological condition than the corresponding area of the right hemisphere.

The patient was too confused to be able to respond correctly in testing for finger-tip number writing perception, so the procedure employed with young children was used in which the subject was required to differentiate only between "X's" and "O's". The patient made 7 mistakes in 20 trials on his right hand and 5 mistakes in 20 trials on his left hand. While these findings, in total, pointed toward some generalized dysfunction, they clearly implicated the right cerebral hemisphere more than the left. The patient also showed definite evidence of constructional dyspraxia in his attempts to copy simple spatial configurations (Figure 3). In drawing the shape of a cross he had some difficulties on the first trial, but these became more prominent and apparent on the second trial. He also demonstrated serious difficulties copying the shape of the key, particularly on the left side of the figure (Figure 4).

In spite of these indications, which up to this point have indicated more serious involvement of the right cerebral hemisphere than the left, the patient also demonstrated pronounced and definite aphasic symptoms which cannot be ignored (Figure 2). When he was asked to spell the word "square" after having named it correctly, he found that he was unable to begin with a letter other than "c." He knew this letter was wrong but he could not correct himself, finally spelling the word "c-q-u-a-r-e." He had similar difficulty spelling "cross," in this instance beginning with "s" and finally, after two attempts, being able to change this to a "c." His best effort, however, was "c-r-o-c-s-s." These indications of confusion in using letters to spell words are obviously not characteristic of poor educational background, but instead represent the type of confusion that is quite characteristic of persons with left cerebral lesions. The patient also had difficulty in spelling "triangle," substituting a "q" for the "g" and recognizing that his effort was incorrect. He demonstrated difficulty even in reading the letters, "MGW," responding "GWM." One might wonder whether he failed to notice the "M" (neglecting the left side of the stimulus configuration) and then noticed it later. However, other aphasic symptoms he demonstrated suggest that he actually is quite seriously confused in dealing with language symbols. There is an element of naming difficulty demonstrated in his reading of the next item. He said, "See the block *fog*," correcting the last word to "dog." He became even more seriously confused on the next reading item as indicated (Figure 2). His difficulties in enunciation seemed to represent principally a tendency toward slurring the words. The basic sound patterns were essentially intact. The patient also seemed to demonstrate evidence of auditory-verbal dysgnosia. He was unable to repeat the sentence "He shouted the warning" correctly, saying the word "morning" instead of "warning." When asked to explain the meaning of the sentence, he was quite confused and the best he was able to do was to say, "Helping? I'd be asking for help, wouldn't I?" It would seem that the patient did not understand the sentence very clearly and had some confusion with respect to decoding of auditory verbal communication. He also showed clear evidence of dyscalculia, not understanding the minus sign and having to ask what it meant. He finally attempted to add and was unable to do this correctly; he then attempted to subtract and again made a mistake. His difficulty in naming was demonstrated when he was shown a key. He called the key "a lock-locker," indicating that he knew what the object was but could not think of the right name. The patient also demonstrated some degree of right-left confusion. In his attempts to write (Figure 3), he demonstrated confusion, particularly on the word "warning." He also spelled "clock" with a "k." These additional instances of confusion in dealing with language symbols would certainly implicate the left cerebral hemisphere. Thus, in addition to the clear evidence of damage to the right cerebral hemisphere, together with lateralizing signs that required postulation of a large lesion in the posterior part of the right cerebral hemisphere, the patient also had clear and definite aphasic symptoms that required postulation of a lesion probably principally located in the left temporal lobe. In our blind interpretation of this case, we felt that the results were quite characteristic of neoplastic involvement, but we raised the possibility of bilateral cerebral metastatic disease, considering the fact that both hemispheres were involved.

NEUROLOGICAL DEFICITS AND EMOTIONAL DIFFICULTIES OF ADJUSTMENT

Many patients show an admixture of neurological and emotional problems. It often is difficult to classify the patient into any of the three categories proposed by Lipowski (17). Some of the changes may be directly related to neuropathological changes, others may be maladaptive manifestations in consideration of other neurological deficits, and some of the changes may be behavioral manifestations stemming merely from the presence of illness. In neuropsychological examination we frequently note instances in which the patient shows deterioration of basic adaptive abilities dependent upon brain functions and also has corresponding problems, depending upon pre-existing personality characteristics and situational factors, that are responses to the illness and directly associated deficits.

We recently examined a 53-year-old farmer with such difficulties and complaints who had completed one year of college. Conventional neurological examination failed to yield any specific abnormalities although a clinical diagnosis of Alzheimer's disease was considered possible. He had been an even-tempered person who had behaved responsibly and performed effectively throughout his life. During the past three years he had noted difficulty with his coordination and he also complained of memory problems. These difficulties had progressed particularly during the year before our examination. The patient said that he now easily becomes "nervous" and in order to accomplish anything he must focus his concentration on the task completely. He said that he sometimes becomes completely confused (his thoughts go "entirely blank") even when dealing with things that are very familiar to him. In an interview with the patient's wife, she indicated that he seemed to have changed emotionally, sometimes being short-tempered even with his grandchildren although he had never previously shown such reactions. Neuropsychological examination was performed at the request of a neurological surgeon in order to obtain additional information with regard to neurological and/or emotional bases for the patient's problems.

The results indicated clearly that his abilities in the past had been well above average. In fact, he presently earned a Verbal IQ that fell in the lower part of the superior range, exceeding about 92% of his age peers. However, his Performance IQ was in the lower part of the normal range, exceeding only 37%. He performed particularly poorly on the Block Design and Digit Symbol subtests. While the overall pattern of subtest scores, considered by itself, did not provide a firm basis for inferring deterioration of cerebral functions, the results on the Wechsler Scale were certainly consistent with such an interpretation. Much more definite results, however, were obtained on Halstead's Tests. The patient earned an Impairment Index of 0.9 (about 90% of the tests in the brain-damaged range), a score that indicated considerably more deterioration of basic adaptive skills than would be expected on an age-related basis. The patient had great difficulty on tasks that required adaptation to novel types of problems or the ability to keep several aspects of the situation in mind at the same time. Thus, his overall efficiency of functioning undoubtedly was seriously compromised. He also showed specific deficits that are indicative of some impairment of brain functions. For example, although measures of lateral dominance showed the patient to be strongly right-handed, right-footed, and right-eyed, his finger-tapping speed was scarcely faster with his preferred than his non-preferred hand. He also showed a definite though mild tendency to fail to perceive tactile stimuli on one side or the other, when stimulation was delivered to both sides simultaneously. He showed other losses of simple abilities related to tactile perception. For example, he made a number of mistakes on both hands in tactile finger localization and in fingertip number writing perception, with the losses being more prominent on the left hand than the right hand in the latter instance. The patient also demonstrated definite evidence of impairment, especially with his left upper extremity, on a complex manipulatory task (Tactual Performance Test). Finally, he showed evidence of serious impairment in his ability to copy simple spatial configurations. The overall set of results, therefore, clearly pointed toward generalized deterioration of cerebral functions. The data were quite convincing in terms of impaired levels of performance, patterns and relationships among the test results, specific deficits of a pathognomonic nature, and impairment in lateralized functioning. Implication of both cerebral hemispheres, without evidence of a specific focal area of involvement in either cerebral hemisphere, constituted a basis for concluding that the patient had some kind of generalized involvement. Our findings, while not permitting a specific diagnosis, were quite compatible with a conclusion of primary neuronal degenerative disease of the brain.

Evaluation of the patient's emotional status constituted another significant approach in understanding his overall problems. He gave evidence of being apprehensive and anxious, doubting his own adequacy in meeting problems in everyday living, having difficulty controlling himself emotionally, and often being annoyed or made angry by minor occurrences. These self-observations on the part of the patient were essentially in agreement with the history information reported above. Further evaluation of the patient indicated that he had distinct depressive tendencies, feelings of personal inadequacy, and a general loss of emotional energy available to apply in order to solve his problems. It would appear that these emotional responses were at least in large part a reaction to the evidence of generalized deterioration of cerebral functions and corresponding impairment of basic adaptive abilities. These findings showed the patient's need for supportive psychotherapy together with realistic training in learning how to disengage from his responsibilities. In essence, he seemed to need to develop an appropriate adjustmental approach geared toward premature retirement. Neglect of the neurological, neuropsychological, or neuropsychiatric aspects of this man's condition would have represented a disservice in terms of the evaluation needed for a complete understanding of his condition.

PSYCHIATRIC DISORDERS AND COGNITIVE IMPAIRMENT

Citation of patients with progressive neurological disease and corresponding emotional problems of adjustment scarcely represents a very complete statement of the contributions to psychiatric evaluation that may be made through neuropsychological examination. In fact, emotional distress in patients with cerebral damage may well represent the rule rather than the exception. Thus, the more significant contribution might very possibly be made in neuropsychologic study of psychiatric rather than neurological patients. Many of these patients have a degree of subtle organic deterioration that undoubtedly is significant with respect to their emotional problems of adjustment. Such patients are observed frequently in the course of neuropsychological evaluation, but detailed and specific studies of the neuropsychological correlates of psychiatric conditions have not yet been performed. We would postulate that particular manifestations of emotional disorder, in fact, may very possibly be determined in part by unique aspects of brain-behavior relationships in the individual patient. Certainly both normal persons and psychiatric patients show individual uniqueness in the behavioral correlates of brain functions. The role of uniqueness in this respect has never been systematically nor thoroughly explored with relation to the development of psychiatric disorders. An approach to this problem may very well represent an outstanding opportunity in developing further insight with respect to psychiatric diagnoses, just as a generation ago neuropsychological evaluation of neurologic patients began to contribute very significantly to developing further understanding of the higher-level aspects of brain functions.

Research Approaches toward Elucidating
Neurological and Psychiatric Interactions

The first approach, obviously, in attempting to relate cerebral damage to indicators of emotional disturbance is to evaluate possible differential effects of cerebral lesions using a standardized measure validated for purposes of expressing emotional disturbances. Dikman did just such a study (2), selecting patients with localized structural cerebral lesions grouped according to both laterality and caudality dimensions, and compared such groups with respect to results obtained on the Minnesota Multiphasic Personality Inventory. In addition to performing statistical evaluations of the Validity scales as well as the Clinical scales using multivariate statistical techniques supplemented by univariate analyses, she also investigated the Anxiety Index (45), the Internalization Ratio (45), the Expressive-Repressive Index (39), the Psychotic Index (11), the Cognitive Slippage Index (19), and the Acting-Out Impulsive Index (7).

While only three studies had previously investigated the MMPI correlates of localized brain lesions involving caudality and laterality dimensions (1, 9, 47), a number of studies had raised a question with respect to the effects of lateralized as well as anterior vs. posterior lesions. Friedman (9) and Williams (47) had reported higher elevations on the psychotic scales of the MMPI for groups with left as compared with right cerebral lesions, but these elevations were not generally significant. However, Hillbom (15) and Flor-Henry (6) had reported a higher incidence of emotional disturbances in patients with left cerebral lesions than patients with right cerebral lesions. On the other hand, Lishman (18) had found patients with right cerebral lesions to be more emotionally disturbed.

More specific reports with respect to differentiation of psychotic disturbances had also been noted. For example Flor-Henry (6), according to clinical evaluation, noted a higher incidence of schizophrenia in patients with left cerebral lesions and manic-depressive psychoses in right hemisphere patients. Studies of this kind, however, must certainly be evaluated with respect to the types of cerebral lesions involved, the methods used for inferring the types of deficits or deviations, and the comparison groups used for drawing specific conclusions. The results of Dikmen (3) did not indicate any special differentiation of MMPI results with respect to cerebral lesion location. Probably the most obvious explanation for these relatively negative results with relation to those previously reported concerns differences in method of personality assessment and the type and unit of behavior studied. While previous results have been based on subjective observations and impressions, Dikmen used an objective method for assessing the degree of deviation from normality. The other studies have used presence vs. absence of symptoms [i.e., apathy, euphoria, anxiety, etc.] (14, 18), or syndromes relating to neurotic or psychotic manifestations (6, 15). It should also be noted that there are differences with respect to the patient population studied and the types of lesions involved; Hécaen used patients with brain tumors, Hillbom and Lishman studied wartime veterans with head injuries, and Flor-Henry restricted his investigation to patients with temporal lobe involvement and psychomotor seizures. Dikman, in contrast, included patients of a diversified nature with tumors, head injuries, and vascular lesions. These various studies have also differed in their use of retrospective neurological information as contrasted with immediately available diagnostic records on each patient included. Finally, Dikmen's studies used methods of data analysis which have become possible only with computer assistance, utilizing a multivariate analog of analysis of variance as contrasted with more simple analytic procedures used by earlier investigators. Thus, while many earlier studies had cited specific emotional components that involved particularly anterior vs. posterior involvement, Dikmen's more objective results do not show such effects. Freeman and Watts (8), for example, have postulated a reduction in anxiety and depression as a result of severance of frontal thalamic tracts (pre-frontal lobotomy), but Dikmen's results do not show any specific MMPI characteristics of frontal lesions. Reitan (35), using a large battery of neuropsychological tests, also failed to show any very striking statistical differences between patients with frontal and nonfrontal lesions.

Thus, it does not appear from the results immediately available that lesions of the left or right cerebral hemisphere, or lesions anteriorly or posteriorly located, have any particular relationship to results obtained on the MMPI. This finding, considered by itself, does not indicate that these various locations of lesions have no relationship to emotional dimensions of response patterns. Instead, the results only indicate that it has not been possible, at the present time, to demonstrate such differential relationships using data based upon MMPI results.

In another study, Dikmen (4) compared two groups of subjects with cerebral lesions, but with all subjects in one of these groups showing evidence of dysphasic difficulties. The groups were comparable with respect to age and education distributions and also with regard to the type of cerebral lesions present, although they obviously were not made comparable with regard to lateralization or location of cerebral lesions. The findings indicated that the presence of aphasia had an influence on personality adjustment as measured by the MMPI. Dikmen cautioned against uncritical transference of interpretations based on psychiatric populations to totally different samples, such as brain-damaged groups with and without aphasia. However, a customary interpretation of the results would lead to a description of the dysphasic group as being more schizoid and having other psychotic tendencies with accompanying thought disturbances. The data would indicate that the dysphasic patients were more impulsive, angry, and possibly psychopathic. On the other hand, some of the findings certainly deviated from any indication of psychotic changes in aphasic patients and it is entirely possible that aphasia, as manifested by results on the MMPI, falls in Lipowski's second category of reactive syndromes related to the problems of coping with the effects of cerebral lesions.

While aphasic patients have been noted to show evidence of depression, irritability, lack of initiative, etc. (46, 40), disturbed affect with ideational disorders has been reported in some stroke patients with severe sensory-motor deficits (44, 16). This type of information raises questions with regard to possible relationships between ability impairment and emotional difficulties. Dikmen was prompted to perform an additional series of studies concerned with the consistency with which emotional reactions occur in combination with particular deficits in persons with brain lesions (2). Using 129 patients with definite neurological diagnoses who also had been administered a very extensive battery of neuropsychological tests (sometimes referred to as the Halstead-Reitan Battery), she was able to compose groups of subjects who showed particular deficits in selected areas. For example, she studied patients with evidence of impairment of verbal intelligence, performance intelligence, concept formation ability, sensory-perceptual skills, motor functions, disparities in verbal as compared with performance intelligence, and disparities in sensory-perceptual as compared with motor functions. The results of these seven studies indicated that persons with cerebral lesions deviated considerably from normals in their MMPI performances. However, there was a striking similarity of profiles across these seven studies with primary elevations on the neurotic scales and secondary elevations on the psychotic scales (especially the Schizophrenia scale). The principal finding, therefore, suggested that brain-damaged patients with different levels of adequacy in adaptive skills behave similarly with respect to emotional responses, including manifestations of depression, worry, and physical complaints.

Differences among the groups with varying patterns of deficits occurred in the degree to which the data imply that subjects are having unusual experiences and interpersonal problems, as shown by higher scores on the psychotic scales. The principal deviation of MMPI results was found in the group with particular and specific impairment of Verbal intelligence, even though results on the Validity scales were within normal limits.

These extensive studies of Dikmen represent a systematized and organized effort to explore emotional problems that may be present in persons with cerebral lesions. While it was important to use a measuring instrument that has been studied in patients with emotional disorders, this aspect of procedure may also have represented a limitation in that responses to individual MMPI items may have different significance among psychiatric patients than among patients with cerebral lesions. It is apparent that this entire area of investigation needs much more detailed and extensive exploration. Conversely, while one can use a psychiatric instrument such as the MMPI to evaluate patients with cerebral lesions, the complementary approach should also be taken. For example, patients classified according to psychiatric categories (rather than neurological findings) should be explored with measures that have been validated with respect to their sensitivity to brain functions. This latter approach, in fact, probably represents one of great value in learning more about the neuropsychological deficits of patients with psychiatric disorders. The neuropsychology of mental illness has never been studied in any great detail but methods are now available and the results that might eventually be obtained could be of very significant value.

REFERENCES

1. Andersen, A. L., & Hanvik, L. J. The psychometric localization of brain lesions: The differential effect of frontal and parietal lesions on MMPI profiles. *Journal of Clinical Psychology*, 1950, 6, 177-180.
2. Dikmen, S. *Minnesota Multiphasic Personality Inventory Correlates of Structural and Functional Cerebral Deficits in Patients with Brain Lesions.* Unpublished doctoral dissertation, University of Washington, 1973.
3. Dikmen, S., & Reitan, R. M. MMPI correlates of localized cerebral lesions. *Perceptual and Motor Skills*, 1974, 39, 831-840.
4. Dikmen, S., & Reitan, R. M. Minnesota Multiphasic Personality Inventory correlates of dysphasic language disturbances. *Journal of Abnormal Psychology*, 1974, 83, 675-679.
5. Engel, W. K., & Meltzer, H. Histochemical abnormalities of skeletal muscle in patients with acute psychoses. Part I. *Science*, 168, 273-276.
6. Flor-Henry, P. Schizophrenic-like reactions and affective psychoses associated with temporal lobe epilepsy: Etiological factors. *American Journal of Psychiatry*, 1969, 126, 148-152.
7. Fordyce, W. Personal communication, January, 1973.

8. Freeman, W., & Watts, J. W. *Psychosurgery: Intelligence, Emotional and Social Behavior following Pre-frontal Lobotomy for Mental Disorders.* Springfield, Ill.: C. C Thomas, 1942.

9. Friedman, S. H. *Psychometric Effects of Frontal and Parietal Lobe Brain Damage.* Unpublished doctoral dissertation, University of Minnesota, 1950.

10. Geschwind, N. The borderland of neurology and psychiatry: Some common misconceptions. In Benson, D. F., and Blumer, D. (Eds.), *Psychiatric Aspects of Neurological Disease.* New York: Grune & Stratton, 1975.

11. Goldberg, L. R. Diagnosticians vs. diagnostic signs: The diagnosis of psychosis vs. neurosis from the MMPI. *Psychological Monographs*, 1965, 79 (Whole No. 602), 1-28.

12. Halstead, W. C. *Brain and Intelligence. A Quantitative Study of the Frontal Lobes.* Chicago: University of Chicago Press, 1947.

13. Haug, J. O. Pneumoencephalographic studies in mental disease. *Acta Psychiatrica Neurologica Scandinavica Suppl.*, 1962, 165, 38, 1-104.

14. Hécaen, H. Mental symptoms associated with tumors of the frontal lobe. In Warren, J. M. and Akert, K. (Eds.), *The Frontal Granular Cortex and Behavior.* New York: McGraw-Hill, 1964.

15. Hillbom, E. Aftereffects of brain injuries. *Acta Psychiatrica Scandinavica*, 1960, Suppl. 142.

16. Horenstein, S. Effects of cerebrovascular disease on personality and emotionality. In Benton, A. L. (Ed.), *Behavioral Change in Cerebrovascular Disease.* New York: Harper & Row, 1970.

17. Lipowski, Z. J. Organic brain syndromes: Overview and classification. In Benson D. F., and Blumer, D. (Eds.), *Psychiatric Aspects of Neurological Disease.* New York: Grune & Stratton, 1975.

18. Lishman, W. A. Brain damage in relation to psychiatric disability after head injury. *British Journal of Psychiatry*, 1968, 114, 373-410.

19. Meehl, P. E., & Dahlstrom, W. G. Objective configural rules for discriminating psychotic from neurotic MMPI profiles. *Journal of Consulting Psychology*, 1960, 24, 375-387.

20. Meltzer, H. Y. Creatine kinase and aldolase in serum: Abnormality common to acute psychoses. *Science*, 1968, 159, 1368-1370.

21. Meltzer, H. Y. Muscle enzyme release in acute psychoses. *Archives of General Psychiatry*, 1969, 21, 102-112.

22. Meltzer, H. Y. Skeletal muscle abnormalities in patients with affective disorders. *Journal of Psychiatric Research*, 1973, 10, 43-57.

23. Meltzer, H. Y. Serum creatine phosphokinase and serum aldolase levels in acutely psychotic patients. In Blume, P., and Freier, E. F. (Eds.), *Enzymology in the Practice of Laboratory Medicine.* New York: Academic Press, 1974.

24. Meltzer, H. Y. Neuromuscular abnormalities in the major mental illnesses. I. Serum enzyme studies. In Freedman, D. X. (Ed.), *The Biology of the Major Psychoses: A Comparative Analysis.* Proceedings of the Association on Research in Nervous and Mental Disease, in press.

25. Meltzer, H. Y., & Crayton, J. W. Subterminal motor nerve abnormalities in psychotic patients. *Nature*, 1974, 249, 373-375.

26. Meltzer, H. Y., & Crayton, J. W. Muscle abnormalities in psychotic patients. II. Serum CPK activity, fiber abnormalities and branching and sprouting of subterminal nerves. *Biological Psychiatry*, 1974, 8, 191-208.

27. Meltzer, H. Y., Elkun, L., & Moline, R. Serum enzyme changes in newly admitted psychiatric patients. *Archives of General Psychiatry*, 1969, 21, 731-738.

28. Meltzer, H. Y., Grinspoon, L., and Shader, R. Serum creatine phosphokinase and

aldolase activities in acute schizophrenic patients and their relatives. *Compreensive Psychiatry*, 1970, 11, 552-558.

29. Meltzer, H. Y., McBride, E., & Poppei, R. W. Rod (memaline) bodies in the skeletal muscle of an acute schizophrenic patient. *Neurology*, 1973, 23, 769-780.

30. Meltzer, H. Y., & Moline, R. Muscle abnormalities in acute psychoses. *Archives of General Psychiatry*, 1970, 23, 481-491.

31. Meltzer, H. Y., Nankin, R., & Raftery, J. Serum creatine phosphokinase activity in newly admitted psychiatric patients. II. *Archives of General Psychiatry*, 1971. 24, 568-572.

32. Mirsky, A. F. Neuropsychological bases of schizophrenia. *Annual Review of Psychology*, 1969, 20, 321-348.

33. Reitan, R. M. An investigation of the validity of Halstead's measures of biological intelligence. *AMA Archives of Neurology and Psychiatry*, 1955, 73, 28-35.

34. Reitan, R. M. The comparative effects of brain damage on the Halstead Impairment Index and the Wechsler-Bellevue Scale. *Journal of Clinical Psychology*, 1959, 15, 281-285.

35. Reitan, R. M. Psychological deficits resulting from cerebral lesions in man. In Warren, J. M. and Akert, K. (Eds.), *The Frontal Granular Cortex and Behavior*. New York: McGraw-Hill, 1964.

36. Reitan, R. M. Psychological changes associated with aging and with cerebral damage. *Mayo Clinic Proceedings*, 1967, 42, 653-673.

37. Reitan, R. M., & Davison, L. A. (Eds.). *Clinical Neuropsychology: Current Status and Applications*. Washington, D.C.: Winston, 1974.

38. Rowland, L. P. Discussion of Meltzer's paper, "Neuromuscular abnormalities in the major mental illnesses." In Freedman, D. X. (Ed.), *The Biology of the Major Psychoses: A Comparative Analysis*. Proceedings of the Association on Research in Nervous and Mental Disease, in press.

39. Sanford, R. N., Webster, H., & Freedman, M. Impulse expression as a variable of personality. *Psychological Monographs*, 1957, 71, (Whole No. 440), 11.

40. Schuell, H., Jenkins, J. J., & Jiménez-Pabón, E. *Aphasia in Adults: Diagnosis, Prognosis and Treatment*. New York: Harper & Row, 1964.

41. Shagass, C. Electrical activity of the brain. In Greenfield, N. S., and Sternbach, R. (Eds.), *Handbook of Psychophysiology*. New York: Holt, Rinehart & Winston, 1972.

42. Slater, E., & Roth, M. (Eds.). *Clinical Psychiatry*. London: Balliére, Tindall & Cassell, 1969.

43. Slater, E., & Glithero, E. A follow-up of patients diagnosed as suffering from "hysteria." *Journal of Psychosomatic Research*, 1969, 9, 9-13.

44. Ullman, M. *Behavioral Changes in Patients following Strokes*. Springfield, Ill.: Charles C Thomas, 1962.

45. Welsh, G. S. An anxiety index and an internalization ratio for the MMPI. *Journal of Consulting Psychology*, 1952, 16, 65-72.

46. Wepman, J. M. *Recovery from Aphasia*. New York: Ronald Press, 1951.

47. Williams, H. L. The development of a caudality scale for the MMPI. *Journal of Clinical Psychology*. 1952, 8, 293-297.

4

The Inadequacies of Contemporary Psychiatric Diagnosis

ROY R. GRINKER, SR., M.D.

In my opinion diagnosis is one of the most important issues confronting modern psychiatry. Diagnoses and classifications cannot be denied as the first scientific steps to answer the question beginning with "what." Without better answers to this question we could not possibly approach or resolve the "how" and "why" questions which bear on causes, course and adaptations to them (26).

The results of earlier attempts at delineation of types of mental illness and the use of a long list of various classifications are no longer adequate (22). For example, here are just a few of the difficulties in diagnostic issues: 1) Many schizophrenics seem to have elevated, excited moods resembling mania. Others are depressed and suicidal, although this mood should be discriminated from anhedonia. We hedge on their labels by diagnosing them neither schizophrenic nor manic-depressive but schizo-affective. There is no evidence from the clinical data that the thought disorders of both are identical, but about 20% of manic-depressives do have some form of thought disorder which is, in my opinion, quite different from the schizophrenic. The notion of one disease which creeps up is frequently not well-founded.

2) There have been attempts to designate acute schizophrenia, with one or several psychotic breakdowns, as a disease different from slowly progressive chronic schizophrenia. This eventually involves what some

69

have called the schizophrenic spectrum which they believe exists in families of index subjects but not in families of acute schizophrenics.

The question of whether or not there is a schizophrenic spectrum is an important issue in current research. Unfortunately Grinker (12) has recently been misquoted as incorporating spectrum types as example of the protean characteristics of schizophrenia. Simply writing about neurotic or psychopathological traits in the families or siblings of index subjects is inadequate because these terms are loosely used and may apply to everyone. Diagnosis and classification require many steps. For example, spectrum concepts would only have validity if genetic markers and specific syndromes could be identified instead of the fragile omnibus term "sick families." Also, the supposed absence of spectrum diagnoses for relatives of acute schizophrenic index cases is not an indication that the acute are genetically unrelated to the other types. Clinicians know that one or several acute breakdowns may precede the development of a chronic and often irreversible course. An attack of acute bronchitis may be the first sign of carcinoma of the lung. The fate of acute schizophrenias can be determined only by a long-term follow-up past age 40.

3) The third issue relates to the changing manifestations of all psychiatric disorders: conversion hysteria, mania, catatonia, hebephrenia, etc. Instead of these diagnostic categories we see more restricted and constricted characters.

4) The issue of diagnosis is also affected by the variability in the life histories of schizophrenics from time to time. The subtypes may shift from one to another, the acute may eventually become chronic, or the chronic may show at least some degree of reversibility even after decades. In this connection we should avoid associating the diagnosis of schizophrenia with other psychoses into which the patient so labeled may slip, since psychoses of toxic, infectious, traumatic, drug, senile, and other origin are also frequently seen in schizophrenics. Most schizophrenics never have an acute psychotic break as it is commonly understood. Nor is recovery from a psychotic break an indication that the process was not a schizophrenia.

There is a voluminous literature on schizophrenia which no one person can completely encompass without the help of a regiment of paid abstractors. What seems clear is that schizophrenia is a system disorder diagnosable by the presence of biopsychosocial parts inefficiently controlled or regulated by an organizational principle. Specific vulnerability, derived from biogenetic factors, is sensitive to a wide variety of precipitating stimuli. Prior to the overt onset, prediction is almost impossible for the premorbid state. Even after a psychotic break or the recognition of thought disorder in a quiescent schizophrenic, prediction of future attacks is very difficult. There are no single causes, and direct relationships between causes and effects have not been established.

The dictionary definition of the term diagnosis indicates a precise and detailed description of the characteristics of an organism for taxonomic classification. Yet the word is derived from the Greek preposition *dia* (apart) and *gnosis* (to perceive or to know). Thus diagnosis in medicine implies the determination of the disease by examination. To discriminate the natures of things requires at the same time distinguishing them from others. The medical profession has the task of naming diseases, following the aphorism that "naming is knowing," which also has the function of excluding diseases not present. The physician understands this well because, in his jargon, he "rules in" and "rules out" possible diagnoses. At least these processes should be part of his formal teaching. Naming and classifying, distinguishing and categorizing, are essential parts of any clinical or research enterprise. The clinician must know what and whom he is treating, in order to decide how to treat. The researcher must know whom he is studying, in order to accumulate comparative knowledge. The issue is not whether we need a means for diagnosis, but whether we can develop to a point where the label and its subtypes will be a valid shorthand, implying specific etiology, symptomatology, prognosis and treatment.

Unfortunately, the "thing out there" or reality is rarely sharply defined, because it is derived both from psychological perception that varies with individual bias, mood, emotional projections, etc.,. and the external environment. The facets of environmental reality and internal constructs constitute an interpenetrating system. There is no neatness to boundaries because the excluded factors are often present as overlapping constituents of one category on another.

It would seem logical that textbooks would accurately portray the necessary symptoms of any syndrome, but these authoritative accounts are often in disagreement about essential and pathognomonic factors. Use of textbooks or monographs alone to insure correct diagnoses is like amateurs painting a picture by the numbers, resulting in a bad imitation of art. How, then, does the clinician make his diagnosis? Certainly not by rote, but by a constant ongoing process of matching concepts and categories with experience.

The clinical psychiatrist uses methods which are complementary: observation of behaviors accurately described; interviews usually in dyadic relations; information from informed sources, usually other members of the patient's family; and psychological test performances. Other ancillary sources of information will be discussed later.

As the psychiatrist interviews, he usually has a memory bank that resonates with the problem under consideration. The better trained, more experienced and older psychiatrists have extensive memories derived from past diagnostic experiences, but no one can attest to their validity.

I first hear and recognize the largest integrated component derived from observation and description of behavior and verbalization. This is like a center piece of a jig-saw puzzle. I then attempt to fit the smaller, not incorporated pieces into this central component. I do not expect that all will fit in and those that do not are extraneous to the essential diagnosis. However, if several large chunks do not fit and seem diametrically opposed to one I have chosen, I then switch to another one as the central piece and attempt to fit the smaller components into it. I may have to do this several times to get the maximum fit from the available bits of information. There can be no unified whole such as the tyro would want, but bits of information related to the individual's personal life and defenses may have to be discarded in order to achieve an ultimate diagnosis. Sometimes this may result in the discarding of important information. For example, some time ago we excluded important data regarding the family as non-essential and annoying pieces (17). Furthermore, only recently have we recognized and given importance to the inherent variability of the schizophrenias (12).

At the present time, the computer is being increasingly utilized; however, although it saves time when large numbers are being studied for research purposes, its reliability is dependent on what the clinician feeds into it from a clinical report and rating system devised by a human being. The computer is not a substitute for the clinician's capacity to probe, elicit and meaningfully report the patient's symptoms in order to derive a syndrome.

Kendall (18) in a recent long-needed monograph agrees that the lost art of diagnosis and classification and the general lack of interest in these areas are the most important issues in contemporary psychiatry, as contrasted with medicine in general where the art of diagnosis as related to therapy and prognosis is not questionsd. There are many definitions of disease categories, all of which are imperfect, but the elements most important are the felt suffering of the patients and their deviant behavior within their society and culture (10). Attempts at accurate diagnosis using purely psychiatric methods of observation, description, questionnaires, rating scales and statistical procedures have not achieved a high degree of *reliability;* there are too many variations of current "bandwagon" fashions, relying on theories, experience, and personality of psychiatrists, all of which lead to biased opinions. Nevertheless, *validity* may be achieved by the use of methods and data from other disciplines and follow-up studies, to verify predictions implicit in every diagnosis.

Who makes the diagnosis? By this time it is well recognized that hospital or clinic records are subject to many distortions. A great variety of persons write these records during different periods when diagnostic rubrics may reflect the fashion of the day, such as the Kohutian "narcissistic neuroses" (20). The teachers, chiefs and attending staff may have a variety of biases. Moreover, many of the hospital records are written by first-year trainees, including, in some centers, clinical psychologists whose training may have been less than relevant to the human problems. Secondly, society's attitudes toward mental illness are altering rapidly in these changing times; tolerance of deviation is higher than in the past. Finally, there has been a decided change in the psychiatric entities, for unknown reasons (13). Manics are fewer, catatonic and hebephrenic schizophrenics are rare, but restricted and constricted character and personality disorders such as the borderline syndrome are increasing, and their diagnostic discrimination is indeed difficult. What all this means is that we appear to have a changing phenomenology in deviant personalities and psychoses. Moreover, articulation with biological, sociological, and cultural systems is not yet possible. I am sure that the changes are not artifacts in diagnosis or labeling, but the how and why are still unknown.

The next question is why make a diagnosis? Why not treat each patient as an individual apart from his diagnosis? The answer is that without diagnosis or categories or typologies we have no science. Perhaps this is what the anti-diagnosis people want—an unscientific, floundering political field in which anyone with empathy, from ward maid to psychiatrist, from concierge to bartender to prostitute, may be equal, and where "encounter" groups of any type may flourish.

To discuss psychiatric problems as problems of living which everyone has does not include the value systems of scientific orientation. It bypasses the decision regarding specific methods of treatment which are ever increasingly dependent on diagnosis. It bypasses the opportunity to predict future course, difficult though that may be. It encourages uniform attitudes to all and decries the active attitude of the traditional physician (4).

The worst part of the arguments of these anti-psychiatrists, who may talk one way but practice another, is their attribution of malignant intent to psychiatry which attempts to treat mental illness, and to prevent suicide and homicide. It attacks the efforts of most psychiatrists who do their best within our state of knowledge and funds, while at the same time these critics behave as the most fascist of our people. During the two world wars, psychiatry attempted to disguise the diagnosis of its victims, first suggesting that they suffered from "shell shock" even though they had never heard a gun fired, then giving them the diagnostic labels "operational fatigue" or "combat fatigue" although they hadn't been near the battle front. This only delayed the mentally ill from obtaining proper treatment. To avoid the so-called pejorative psychiatric labels of diagnosis by calling them problems of living which are universal is to abrogate the help a psychiatrist may give.

The recent deluge of books and articles asserting that mental illness is a myth, written in unscientific, intemperate language designed to appeal to far-right political sectors of the population, is not responsible for psychiatry's weak diagnostic approaches. However, it does require some response that will not elevate the proponents of "myth" to a position worthy of debate, which Moore (23) has done in a lengthy philosophical discussion.

Even though mental illness has no specific referent in our language, it is not therefore an unscientific concept. The task is to define as accurately as possible the *what* of illness in suitable terms. How we do this will be considered later.

The recent intense interest in differentiating the medical model from "problems in living" models does not indicate a commitment to understanding, but rather represents 1) a pragmatic approach for the nonmedical psychotherapists, and 2) the extreme human rights advocates who contend that psychiatrists have no role as agents of society. They suggest that psychiatrists, unlike physicians involved in treating infectious and contagious diseases, should not be permitted to isolate the destructive and self-destructive psychotic.

The psychological system has no specific morphological structure, but represents a structure or structures in the sense of consistent patterns of function; with other parts (biogenetics, physiology, biochemistry, life experiences, hormonal, etc) it helps constitute a system. Unfortunately, at least one so-called structure has been reified. The ego is a concept that can be in conflict only in the abstract. It functions through a "self" in behaviors. It is hypothesized that these are behavioral-action models utilizing somatic sources of energy, not some vague "psychic energy." Behaviors feed back in various ways before and after action to result in a variety of alterations in affect and cognition.

The "ego" together with other terms results in a jargon not universally defined inside or outside the specialty of psychoanalysis. Words are strung together, piled on as it were, for the purposes of explanation, often misidentified as causes (19). But more and more words end up meaning less and less. Such strange language weakens diagnoses of categories, syndromes, causes, and adaptational benefits. They only serve to give to some a false sense of erudition and omniscience, and thwart serious attempts at diagnosis and classification.

"Whether we are viewing categories of mental illness or mental health, or for that matter, any living process, each constitutes a large field containing a large number of variables the permutations of which enable us to observe combinations and recombinations that determine types or subcategories. How to do this is the problem. The process perspective eventually requires operational definitions" (10).

Of these, two are invariable: 1) the biogenetic component and 2) the social and cultural environments. The developmental variants from infancy to the dedifferentiation of the aged are highly individualized. But as Weiss (25) states: "The component parts when operating in the common integral system are interdependent in such a manner that as any one of them strays off the norm in one direction, this entails an automatic counteraction of the others. This is the principle of homeostasis, whether based on circuitry of electrical controls, enzymatic feedback, or intrapsychic informational processes."

Anna Freud (8) stated: "Even supposing that we have complete knowledge of the etiological factors that decide a given result, nevertheless what we know about them is only their quality, not their relative strengths. Some of them are suppressed by others because they are too weak and they therefore do not affect the final result. But we never know beforehand which of the determining factors will prove the weaker or the stronger." As a result concurrent independent psychological techniques, objective measurement and prediction require follow-up studies to determine which changes occur spontaneously or as a result of treatment. All together these constitute what we call validity.

In sum, normality and illness are only polarities of a wide range of integrations; without any strains (an unlikely hypothetical condition), there is only normality. When strained, the organismic systems respond according to the processes by which the many subsystems have become integrated. There are no new defenses or coping devices—they have already been built into the organism. Thus, the degree of health or illness in the stress responses reveals the quality and quantity of integration. But the boundaries between health and illness in all of medicine, particularly psychiatry, are not sharp. Yet most psychiatrists do adhere to the medical model, using biological plus psychological and behavioral data to reach a diagnosis.

In separating the practice of clinical psychiatry from psychiatry as a science, we are dealing with a weak dichotomy because clinical psychiatry can be approached scientifically and the sciences that form the system of scientific psychiatry are ultimately concerned with operational deviations in human behavior and require clinical contact and expertise in eliciting behavioral, cognitive and affective data. The data of the basic sciences and those at the psychological level supplement each other. Unfortunately life histories of patients reveal considerable diversity and general principles are difficult to abstract. In other words, it is difficult to separate what is individual and incidental from what is general and essential, thus making a system of classification extremely difficult.

The stages or phases of development may be viewed from a variety of theoretical positions: psychosexual, epigenetic, behavioral, or learning theories. They all have in common the concept of primary undifferentiation, gradually passing through critical periods of differentiation which are age-specific. All include concepts of process not only in differentiation, but in the phenomenon of dedifferentiation. For each phase there are specific scientific disciplines concerned with creating and storing knowledge, specific medical specialties for diagnosis and therapy, and specific psychotherapeutic strategies, as well as corresponding social institutions (9).

During the last several decades clinical psychiatric research has become much more sophisticated through the use of detailed, especially constructed interviews, observations of behavior, questionnaires, psychological tests, and follow-back or follow-up studies put together by appropriate rating scales and computer analyses. Improved statistical techniques called cluster analysis, discriminate analysis, principal component analysis, and factoring have successfully dealt with quantitative scales in a way vastly more productive than simple scanning or one-to-one correlations.

Yet psychiatrists have not overcome their anachronistic concepts of dichotomies (14) based on the kind of "yes or no" or "night or day" thinking more appropriate to digital computers than to clinical explorations. We still read and hear of medical versus social models of the mind, of nature versus nurture, of reductionism versus humanism in psychiatry. We still hear about endogenous versus exogenous, and process versus reactionary schizophrenia. In the affective sphere, anger is considered in or out, depressions are either monopolar or bipolar. In the complicated field of schizophrenia, the acute form is considered by some as a separate disease, not precedent to or part of the phases of the chronic form (2).

The use of either-or, of so-called psychological structures and states, is a remnant of outmoded thinking that is apparently difficult to abandon. This also applies to our defective Diagnostic and Statistical Manual of Mental Disorders. Indeed, even complementarity, as, for example, heavy biogenetic preparation requiring low degrees of stress and weak hereditary factors requiring high degrees of stress to produce overt disease, has not completely superseded the concept of single causes in linear effects.

A systems or unitary approach to psychiatry, which is better suited to its use, cannot succeed when parts of the biopsychosocial system are considered to be structuralized in fixed points as states. This does not express a dynamic process in action, functioning as part of multiple causes leading to types of unhealthy disturbances or to a variety of forms of adaptation, defenses, and coping processes (15).

Not only do we need to clarify and develop a consensus regarding the gross diagnostic categories, but we need to develop classifications into subtypes necessary for different forms of treatment and more accurate prognosis. Our experiences with the borderline syndrome may serve as an example (11). Our research design was based on objectively observable behavior, which we then rated in terms of traits derived from the point of view of ego-psychology. We made the assumption that objective behavior observed and quantified over a sufficient period of time would be a valid sample of a particular individual's behavior and hence ego-function. Furthermore, the accumulation of such data for a large number of similarly designated patients would result in a sharper definition of that specific diagnostic category.

The information from this group was combined with an older age group from a previous study. Four discrete groups of patients emerged from the combined sample, but a cluster analysis gave a close association between two groups of two. In one pair of these groups there is still hope of meaningful relationships for the subjects who are either angry at the world or are passive and compliant. In the other pairing of groups there is a preponderant lack of self identity associated with depressive loneliness.

When we use behaviors for diagnosis (6), including verbal and global behaviors plus feelings and social competence focusing on the "here and now," we omit the past, namely, biogenic, early experiential, precipitating factors, salutary and destructive life influences, and current social and cultural criteria. To make a complete diagnosis using these factors we require a multidisciplinary research team (a basic methodology in all humanist behavioral sciences), because each element needs the expertise of another discipline. Science thus requires a systems approach, all specialists utilizing the same subjects as close in time as possible. Thereby we avoid the biases in empirical studies that tend to conform to the theory of individual disciplines.

The psychiatrist can observe, describe, rate, test for reliability based on exact definitions of traits, expose his results to studies of validity, and convert his data into statistical analyses which ultimately depend on the primary empirical studies. These are safeguarded by repetitive examination and by a long-term follow-up. Even then he needs controls consisting of other entities and healthy subjects.

The procedure most likely to be of value is the follow-up. The follow-up is fraught with difficulties which can, however, be overcome. There is a high attrition rate of patients moving to unknown areas, suicide, death from other causes, reluctance to opening up a painful area, etc. It requires the use of an out-patient clinic, beds for rehospitalization, and re-interviews and ratings by the same psychiatrists who first performed these functions.

Provided that life events are sufficiently taken into consideration, it is my belief that the best outcome data would result from comparison groups composed of hospitalized patients and healthy subjects over a period of

15 to 20 years or until subjects reach age 40. It is only then that we will be able to answer the "what" question of categories and subtypes.

The diagnostic dilemma has revolved in circles for more than a century although the shifts have different sequences. The history of psychiatry presented by Alexander and Selesnick (1) clearly indicates how feelings and attitudes toward the deviances of behavior and their treatments reflect the value systems and ethics of the contemporary culture. Even the development of modern science is a value component of contemporary culture.

Psychiatry has become recognized as a conglomerate of many sciences. All of these ultimately focus on human mental problems which may require systems of evaluation based on diagnostic accuracy, rating scales, statistical reliability, and efforts at validation.

In addition, the component sciences of psychiatry, such as biogenetics, neurochemistry, endocrinology, and neurophysiology, as well as information, communication and perceptual psychology, combined with the social sciences, offered new insights into the systems of cause, course and outcome which transcended dynamic psychology. All of these disciplines utilize the language of behaviors. It became apparent that the many-sided, multifactorial, psychosomatic, systems approaches which include motivational or dynamic sub-systems only as a part require a basic sense of commonality of what is being studied (3). Our greatest task at present is to develop bridging methods and data. If we dodge the issue that there are categories of mental disturbances with specific course and prognosis, we have no science. There can be no scientific therapy without clinical categories as guidelines to facilitate the study of the life-history of specific disturbances, their spontaneous course, and the interrelationships among causative factors.

~ The scientific attitude is characterized by curiosity expressed in the form of three questions: What, How and Why? The order of these questions is important since causes (*How*) and purposes (*Why*) are not understandable unless we know *What* we are studying or talking about. Paul Meehl (21), a distinguished psychologist, critically states: "Rather than decrying nosology, we should become masters of it, recognizing that some of our psychiatric colleagues have in recent times become careless and even unskilled in the art of formal diagnosis."

The hitch in diagnoses is not only in definition but in the exclusion of much data, even among pure clinicians. The dynamic school overlooks much of behavior, while the behaviorally oriented school ignores large hunks of data about feelings and concerns. Both have a tendency to overlook other systems of data which are becoming increasingly available and valid. Psychodiagnosis in one- to two-hour sessions may be a brilliant narcissistic exercise for the professor to astound his students, but we know the results are not impressive over the long run. Criticisms of diagnostic reliability, and hence usefulness, should not result in abandoning the process, but should lead to inclusion of extended areas of information requiring much more time than an interview and/or conference. Indeed, one of the most disquieting problems is the difference between the English and American diagnoses of schizophrenia even with each using the same information (5).

Good diagnostic systems require unbiased theoretical orientations, simplicity, reliability and consistency over time, and acceptability in relation to processes that can elicit traits [such as interviewing technique, comprehensiveness and culture-free criteria (4)]. The clinician uses any one or all of these sources that are available to him. His diagnostic acumen is based on his capacity to utilize the essence from all sources with which to build a gestalt that is characteristic of a symptom-complex or syndrome currently generally recognized and labeled.

However, such a technique does not suffice as a method for scientific studies, for example, to delineate a new category or to develop subcategories or typologies. In general, scientific information is obtained by collecting observations and measurements under specific conditions, encoding the data in terms characteristic of the statistical model to be used, processing the data, and checking the results again against the original events. Royce (24) exemplifies this in terms applicable to clinical research: 1) standard conditions of observations as on a nursing unit, 2) under specified conditions even though the variables are not controlled, 3) by many persons, 4) observing specified variables, 5) with repetitive observations, and 6) statistical analyses leading to the determination of the contribution of each variable. To this we must add the checking of results for their logical relationship with clinical experience.

Whenever we use such terms as holistic, process, or global, we become satisfied, sense closure, and flee from the operational. Empirical research requires the observation of symptoms, behaviors, or functions, but these are far from fundamental causes. The sociologist looks outward to the social world of experience with his special techniques. The psychologist looks inward at processes that he terms intervening variables, and the biologist, all too frequently reductionistic, searches for genic, biochemical or physiological deficits. Yet each focus constitutes a transacting part of the larger field from which hypothetical constructs or theory may be developed and tested. Actually, a nosological and classificatory focus of the interdisciplinary components of psychiatry may facilitate their articulation.

In our quest for certainty, however, we have almost automatically forced natural phenomena and the laws pertaining to them into the straitjacket of continuity. We tend to close the arc of open circles and demand universal laws because of our abhorrence of discontinuities, belying our empirical information; thus, our concepts become comfortably uniform. This may be one of the reasons why some psychiatrists obliterate obvious differences and try to make of all psychopathology one disease.

How can we classify psychiatric illness? Certainly not by means of symptoms (more easily by syndromes) and not by isolated etiological factors that exclude all others (16). Ideally, diagnoses can be made only after an exhaustive search for all possible contributing etiological factors (7). This requires too much time and expense, and also delays the scientific purposes of diagnostic classification: to enable a wide variety of disciplines to study the "what," to test a wide variety of treatments, including natural spontaneous course, and to determine the life history to the final end. In the meantime, we should abstain from diagnostic nihilism, grand holistic generalizations, and minute classifications.

What we can state, for example, when the schizophrenic organization weakens or breaks is that there are two classes of symptoms as originally formulated by Hughlings Jackson. One is the loss of functional control determined by the absence of high level thinking and feeling. These weak or deficient parts often cannot be compensated for by other functions. The other is the presence of old functions, always alive but repressed or controlled, revived by the absence or weakness of regulation.

Finally, another diagnostic issue concerns the adaptive or so-called restitutive functions attempting to cover up the lost functions or the revived functions of the schizophrenic process. Adaptation is often successful and no further difficulties ensue. A short-term outcome is not definitive.

A systems approach takes into account several conceptual models such as the constitutional, concerned with structure and function; the integrative processes and resistances against disintegration; and determinants that disclose the functions and purposes of the whole in transactions with other systems. Thus, sophisticated theories or operations are multivariate rather than two-variable or linear cause and effect. Multiple observers at different positions are needed.

Psychopathology, therefore, is a system disturbance, and not loss of a single function. It is only by viewing psychopathology in this manner as a system that we can establish diagnostic criteria and analyze the "what." We need to compare what we call pathology with what our society and culture conceive as healthy, with the degree of dissolution, the age specific behaviors, the time course of the syndrome (follow-up), and the response to various therapies.

If we consider ourselves as humanists who are devoted to concerned care of our patients (as all good physicians should) and approach any category of behavior deviance as psychotherapists, we should hope for better understanding of the human condition under stress. In truth, we require a sound systems approach, multidisciplinary consciences if not operations, and the capacity to endure contemporary uncertainty in order to arrive eventually at a better concept of growth, differentiation, and disease.

REFERENCES

1. Alexander, F. G., & Selesnick, S. T. *The History of Psychiatry*. New York: Harper and Row, 1966.
2. Bellak, L. (Ed.). *Schizophrenia: A Review of the Syndrome*. New York: Grune and Stratton, 1969.
3. Bertalanffy, L., von. *General Systems Theory*. New York: George Braziller, 1968.
4. Cohen, E. S., Harbin, H. T., & Wright, M. J. Some considerations in the formulation of psychiatric diagnosis. *Journal Nervous and Mental Diseases*, 160, 422-428, 1975.
5. Cooper, J. *Psychiatric Diagnosis in New York and London*. London: Oxford, 1972.
6. Eron, L. D. *The Classification of Behavior Disorders*. Chicago: Aldine Printing Co., 1960.
7. Fowler, D. R., & Langsbaugh, R. J. The problem-oriented record. *Archives of General Psychiatry*, 32, 831-834, 1975.
8. Freud, A. *The Ego and the Mechanisms of Defense*. New York: Int. Universities Press, 1946.
9. Grinker, R. R., Sr. Normality viewed as a system. *Archives of General Psychiatry*, 17, 320-324, 1967.
10. Grinker, R. R., Sr., & Nunnally, J. C. The phenomena of depression. In Katz, M. M., Cole, J. O., and Barton, W. E. (Eds.), *Role and Methodology of Classification in Psychiatry and Psychopathology*, pp. 249-261, 1967.
11. Grinker, R. R., Werble, B., & Drye, R. C. *The Borderline Syndrome*. New York: Basic Books, 1968.
12. Grinker, R. R., Sr. Diagnosis and schizophrenia. In Cancro, R. (Ed.), *The Schizophrenic Reactions*, pp. 59-69, 89-92. New York: Brunner/Mazel, 1970.
13. Grinker, R. R., Sr. Changing styles in psychiatric syndromes. *American Journal Psychiatry*, 130, 151-152, 1973.

14. Grinker, R. R., Sr. Dichotomies, states and structures. *American Journal Psychiatry*, 132:739-740, 1975.
15. Grinker, R. R., Sr. The relevance of general systems theory to psychiatry. In Arieti, S. (Ed.), *The American Handbook of Psychiatry*, 2nd edition, Vol. 6. New York: Basic Books, 1975.
16. Kaplan, A. *The Conduct of Inquiry*. San Francisco: Chandler Printing Co., 1964.
17. Katz, M. et al. Influence of symptom perception, past experience, and ethnic background on diagnostic decisions. *American Journal Psychiatry*, 125, 937-947, 1969.
18. Kendall, R. E. *The Role of Diagnosis in Psychiatry*. Oxford-London: Blackwell Scientific Publications, 1975.
19. Kernberg, O. *Borderline Conditions and Pathological Narcissism*. New York: Jason Aronson, 1975.
20. Kohut, H. *The Analysis of the Self*. New York: Int. Universities Press, 1971.
21. Meehl, P. E. Some rumination on the validation of clinical procedures. *Canadian Journal of Psychology*, 13, 102-128, 1959.
22. Menninger, K., et al. *The Vital Balance*. New York: Viking, 1963.
23. Moore, M. S. Some myths about "Mental Illness." *Archives of General Psychiatry*, 32, 1483-1500, 1975.
24. Royce, J. R. *Psychology and the Symbol*. New York: Random House, 1965.
25. Weiss, P. The cell as a unit. *Journal of Theoretical Biology*, 5, 389-397, 1963.
26. Zubin, J. Classification of the behavior disorders. *Annual Review of Psychology*, 18, 373-401, 1967.

5

The Limits of Standardisation

JOHN K. WING, M.D., PH.D.

INTRODUCTION

I shall be concerned, in this paper, with the development of techniques of making the processes of psychiatric diagnosis more reliable and communicable. Such techniques have recently had a good deal of success, but this has only been achieved by laying down specific limits, outside which they are not applicable. A consideration of these limits will not only allow a summary of progress to date but also provide an opportunity to discuss the points at which they might be extended. We shall thus be working from the known towards the unknown.

The paper will be based mainly upon one particular set of techniques, which has been under development and test for some 15 years, but this will also provide an opportunity for broader comment. I should like to begin by considering the way our concepts of illness have developed.

THE DEVELOPMENT OF CONCEPTS OF DISEASE

When we examine the history of medicine, and even more the history of psychiatry, it is plain that science, in the sense of a systematic trial and error approach to problem solving through the rational elimination of error, has only recently become influential. When members of the "little savage tribes" described by Lévi-Strauss try to understand the various misfortunes that befall them, they do not require as many different types of explanation as people in western industrial societies. Crops may fail, babies may die, a man in the village may steal from his neighbours, another may run amok, a woman may develop hideous sores. Environmental disasters, physical handicaps, personal distress, socially undesirable behaviour, and madness can all be seen as the result of intervention in human affairs by supernatural forces. Such an infinitely flexible system of explanation requires interpreters. Morris Carstairs (9) found that villagers in Northern India lost belief in his powers as a healer when he asked them about their symptoms:

> in their eyes, a healer who lacker the ability to *know* these things by virtue of his supernatural gifts was scarcely likely to be able to contend with the spiritual cause of their complaint. . . . It became plain that the great majority of remedies which I saw deployed were, physiologically speaking, quite irrelevant to the disease process itself. Instead, they were designed to bolster the morale of the patient and his family, and their effectiveness depended upon the authority and conviction which they imparted.

The western doctor is here distinguishing between two different types of theory, both of which, at the point of application, are psychosomatic. His own is based upon a knowledge of "physiology" and the ways in which, when it goes wrong, various "disease processes" may be produced. Each of these processes gives rise to recognizable patterns of complaint that can be matched against the complaints of individual patients, in order to suggest what remedies should be prescribed. The theories of the native healer are more diffuse but they, too, have developed by a slow and unsystematic process of trial and error and have, in practice, their own kind of success. F. E. Clements described several types of theory used by primitive tribes, each of which gave rise to a type of treatment. The theory of spirit possession, for example, suggests treatment by exorcism, by mechanical extraction of the foreign spirit, or by transferring it to some other object or being. The theory of sorcery suggests treatment by counter-magic (14).

The difference between the scientific concept and the social attribution of disease is well illustrated by the South American tribe described by Dubos (13), in which a disfiguring disease, dyschromic spirochaetosis, characterized by multicoloured spots on the skin, was so common that those who did *not* have it were regarded as abnormal and excluded from marriage. Dyschromic spirochaetosis is a serious disease, recognizable at once to any expert, but only those who had it were thought to be healthy.

All of us are exposed, from early childhood, to old wives' tales and folk beliefs that are not dissimilar to the magical explanations commonly adopted by such peoples. The modern professional has inherited something of the mystery and charisma of the earlier religious healers and prophets, and naturally all doctors have acquired, during their early years, the beliefs about health that are current in their own society. The history of medicine is full of examples of ingenious but almost completely false theories about various ills and their treatments, put forward in pseudo-scientific guise by qualified medical practitioners. H. T. Pledge (29) suggested that this tendency reached its climax in eighteenth century Europe, and that thereafter it was increasingly the province of quacks.

> One of these ideas was the very simple one of John Brown of Edinburgh, that all ills are either depressions or excitements; to be treated, respectively, with alcohol or opium. His own ills were depressions and he died of the cure.

The development of scientific medicine occurred against a background of folk belief and ingrained social attitudes as to what constituted health and deviance from health. The formulation that certain patterns of mental and bodily change were explicable in terms of specific and testable disease theories depended a great deal on what was regarded as socially undesirable. It could be argued theoretically that great musical or mathematical ability is inherited, at least potentially, and that it will one day be possible to recognize which people have such abilities by measuring the activity of certain parts of the brain. There are the elements here of a disease theory; however, because few societies are likely to regard musical or mathematical genius as undesirable, it is most improbable, though not impossible, that either will ever be called a disease. The term "social deviation" has something of the same bias. The scientific approach does not vary whether we are investigating genius or jaundice, only the label changes. But whether we call the trait an "ability" or a "disability" depends mostly upon social norms.

J. R. Baker (3) gives a splendid example of this process in his discussion of ethnic differences in endogenous body-odour. People with an acute sense of smell are aware of differences in the quality and intensity of axillary odour, which may vary between individuals, and in the same individual at different times (for example, in relation to the menstrual cycle). In general, Europeans and Negroes are smelly, whereas most Japanese are not. The latter are therefore very sensitive to axillary odour and almost have a horror of it. However, 10% of Japanese do have smelly armpits just like Europeans, possibly because they have Ainu ancestry. (The Ainu are of the same ethnic type as Europeans.) "The existence of the odour is regarded among Japanese as a disease, *osmidrosis axillae,* which used to warrant exemption from military service. Certain doctors specialize in its treatment, and sufferers are accustomed to enter hospital."

Clearly, the development of disease theories is part of a process of scientific investigation but, at the same time, there are powerful social forces influencing which characteristics should be investigated in this way. As in other fields of human endeavour, medical theories and techniques gradually become more refined; some are found more useful in explaining and relieving socially recognized disability than others. This progress is achieved at the expense of accepting that only certain problems are amenable to the new ideas, while the mass of amorphous complaints about deviance or ill-health have to be left to more traditional explanations or to agnosticism. On the one hand, there is still a tradition in medicine that treats loss of morale independently of cause, and this can be quite useful. On the other hand, scientific medicine has achieved its success by concentrating on more and more specific problems. The most developed disease theories are based on a knowledge of the homeostatic mechanisms that maintain some relevant bodily function, such as blood sugar, within known limits. When specific causal effects operate, one or more than one normal cycle becomes unbalanced, the limits are exceeded, and a chemical syndrome such as diabetes mellitus becomes manifest.

Therefore, to put forward a diagnosis is, first of all, to recognise a condition, and then to put forward a theory about it. Theories are meant to be tested.

The most obvious test is whether applying the theory is helpful to the patient. Does it accurately predict a form of treatment that reduces disability without leading to harmful side-effects? Does it give some idea of the future course and outcome? At the very least, can the sufferer or the relatives be given the consolation that there are other people with the same condition, that it has a name, and that there are ways of coping with it? A further use of a disease theory is less obvious but in some ways just as important. It can lead to the acquisition of new information, for example concerning pathology, physiology and aetiology. This may not be of immediate benefit to any one individual, but it may lead to discoveries that will suggest future means of treatment or prevention and add to the store of potentially useful knowledge.

Thus there are two essential components to any disease concept. The first is the recognition of a syndrome; the second is the construction of an explanatory theory, which may be purely academic at the time it is first put forward, but which may also be of value in application. In the rest of this paper I shall be mainly concerned with the first of these components and with the uses and limitations of standardisation. I have dealt with explanatory theories and their validation elsewhere (45) and other papers in this symposium are largely concerned with them. I will simply state here that, unless it is possible to recognise disease syndromes reliably, it is very difficult to test theories about them. It has become clear that a high degree of communicability among clinicians can be achieved and is worth achieving, and that even some of the well-publicised differences between some American and some European psychiatrists can, in large measure, be understood and used as a basis for advance towards a common language. Clinicians in different parts of the world are learning to speak to each other in mutually comprehensible terms (43). I hope to show that simply improving the techniques of recognising and classifying psychiatric disorders can raise important scientific problems and that, by making comparisons possible, it can also do much to improve our means of testing theories.

The attitude of critical curiosity implicit in this approach is well illustrated by the limerick about the Crusader's wife.

> *A Crusader's young wife from the garrison*
> *Spent a couple of nights with a Saracen.*
> *She was not over-sexed,*
> *Or jealous, or vexed;*
> *She just wanted to make a comparison.*

DEFINING AND NAMING SYMPTOMS AND SYNDROMES

Sydenham laid down three criteria for the recognition of a disease syndrome: that a group of symptoms should be intercorrelated amongst themselves, should be differentiable from other syndromes, and should possess a characteristic pattern over time. We have seen that the process of recognition is sometimes a very long one, but it can also be the result of a flash of clinical insight. Aretaeus described a "melting of the flesh and limbs to urine" followed by early death, and named the syndrome "diabetes." The naming, or (in modern terms) labeling, can be as important as the recognition. Both Haslam (20) and Itard (23) described, with brilliance and clarity, single cases of early childhood autism. But it was not until Kanner (24) not only matched the creativity of their recognition and the clinical precision of their description of the syndrome, but actually gave it a name, that it became clear how different the condition was from mental retardation, or schizophrenia, or the other conditions with which it had hitherto been lumped. Kanner based his description on 11 children. That was enough. Large numbers and a sophisticated statistical analysis are not necessary for all advances in psychiatry.

The present generation of psychiatrists stands on the shoulders of its predecessors. Anyone who tries to standardise the processes underlying diagnosis must begin by defining symptoms and syndromes that have already been recognised and described by countless others. The best descriptions for the purpose are based directly on the experiences described by patients, with no interpolation or interpretation by the clinician. A glossary of definitions must lie at the heart of any standardised system. The ninth edition of the Present State Examination (PSE), for example, consists of 140 items, each of which is defined in the glossary (49). Without such a glossary, it is impossible to be sure that users mean the same thing by a symptom such as depersonalisation, for example, and impossible to try to train people, in a practicably brief time, to use the system. It is also difficult totally to standardise a method of examination designed to foster the differential recognition of the selected symptoms. A technique such as the PSE is based on the assumption that the examiner knows what he is looking for. His own previous experience and training are therefore extremely important.

The process of rating involves several kinds of decision. The first, and most important, is whether the symptom is absent: rated 0. The second is the degree of severity, if it is present: rated 1 or 2. Other options are "not known" or "not applicable." The first two decisions have to be taken by clinicians every time they undertake a psychiatric examination. Guiding criteria are laid down for both types of decision in the PSE glossary, all based on clinical experience. These basic considerations determine the form of the PSE schedule, which is that of a list of 140 items, most representing familiar psychiatric symptoms, each defined in the glossary, and each of which can be rated absent, present in moderate degree, or present in severe degree.

If the purpose of the examination and the definitions of symptoms are well known, the way the interview is conducted is relatively less important, although it is still necessary to introduce a degree of structure. This is done by adopting a number of well-known devices already used by clinicians when conducting a diagnostic interview. The individual is first given an opportunity to describe the experiences that have particularly bothered him or her during the previous month, then the examiner either begins the systematic review in the order laid down or, if the individual clearly wishes to describe some particular group of symptoms first, begins with that. The examiner is free at any time to revert to a section that has already been covered, or to move to another area, even though it does not follow the order suggested in the schedule. Similarly, a form of questioning is laid down but the clinician is not bound to adopt it. The technique of interview is based upon "cross-examination"; that is, the individual is asked to describe experiences and the examiner then asks sufficient further questions to establish, to his own satisfaction, whether the symptom is present. The fact that a subject says "Yes" to a question, about anxiety for example, is not taken as sufficient evidence that the symptom is present. The subject must describe the experience in terms that the examiner recognises as compatible with the definition given in the glossary; otherwise the symptom is rated as absent (or, occasionally, as "not known"). Another clinical device incorporated into the interview is the use of the cut-off point. If the examiner is satisfied, on the basis of the answers to certain obligatory questions, that no symptoms of that type are present, the questions below the cut-off point need not be asked. But again, this requires a deliberate decision by the examiner.

Thus, a Present State Examination, carried out by a trained and competent clinician, should not sound like a standard procedure at all, but much like an ordinary clinical interview. This degree of skill is, of course, achieved only after a great deal of experience. Beginners have to stay quite close to the procedure laid down. All appearances to the contrary, the rating of symptoms using these techniques is reasonably reliable.

Some psychiatrists, however, do not wish to use such directive techniques, and they cannot use the system.

The output from the examination is a symptom-profile composed of 140 ratings, all positive ratings being illustrated by narrative descriptions in the subject's words. The next step is to condense the symptoms into syndromes. This can be done on the basis of clinical experience or on the basis of statistical clustering techniques. It is at this point that a fact, implicit in everything that has been said hitherto, has to be made explicit: *Clinical decisions are always based upon theory.* No choice of a symptom, a definition, a form of questioning, a cut-off point, or a rating, can be made in a clinical vacuum. Purely statistical clustering also involves assumptions, but these are not clinical in nature. The most obvious, and also, in my opinion, the most fallacious, is that each item put into the statistical melting pot can be regarded as equal in weight to all the others. This goes clean against all clinical experience. It is rather like assuming that a score, formed from summing the ratings on all PSE symptoms, from worrying to thought insertion, can be used instead of a diagnosis. In fact, clinicians always use a hierarchy of diagnostic importance, and any statistical clustering must be judged against this.

PSE syndromes therefore have a mixed clinical and statistical basis (41, 49). Even where two syndromes are strongly associated together statistically and both are differentiated from other syndromes, as is the case with syndromes (NS) and (AH), they are kept separate in the Syndrome Check List if diagnostic considerations require it (49). In this particular case, syndrome (NS) is composed of symptoms described by Kurt Schneider (33) as being of "the first rank" for the recognition of schizophrenia. Syndrome (AH) consists of voices experienced as speaking *to* the patient, which are not regarded as first rank symptoms by Schneider, because they can occur in mania and in the psychotic form of depressive disorder. In earlier studies it was indeed found that syndrome (AH) occurred in these disorders, though rarely. Appropriate changes in the definition of symptoms have allowed a differentiation to be made on the basis of content, with the result that syndrome (AH) is now found almost exclusively in schizophrenic disorders (32, 51, 52). If this is found to hold true in further studies, the two syndromes could be combined. Meanwhile, no harm is done by keeping them separate. In the long run, statistical and clinical criteria of definition have to come together. The major advantage of the present PSE syndromes is that they do not cut across current diagnostic classifications, even though each meets minimal statistical standards. They also provide a useful descriptive summary of current mental state, since a profile of 38 syndromes is more easily comprehended than a profile of 140 symptoms.

It may reasonably be claimed that the first two of Sydenham's criteria for the recognition of syndromes can be met by using standard techniques. The third, a characteristic pattern over time, will be considered later.

Classification into "Disorders"

The term "classification" can be used in two ways, to mean the system of classes into which objects or data are sorted and the process of allocating each object or datum to a class. Hempel (21) suggests that an ideal classification in the first sense should be mutually exclusive and jointly exhaustive; that is, each object should be allocated to one class and one class only, and a class should be available for each object, ensuring a minimum of uncertainty and ambiguity.

Several types of information may be required for a diagnostic classification that cannot be derived from a present state examination: in particular, information from past episodes of disorder, information from pathological investigations, and information concerning various possible aetiological factors. The simplest case, in which the clinical examination contains all the information required, can be considered first. This is likely to be true of the disorders suffered by patients recently admitted to hospital with one of the functional psychoses or neuroses. The principles of the CATEGO program, which incorporates a set of classifying rules based on clinical experience, specified with sufficient precision to be applied by computer to any individual profile of PSE symptoms, have been described in detail and need not be repeated here. The most important principle, however, does bear repetition. This is that psychiatric classification is hierarchical in nature (17, 41, 49). This principle is familiar to all clinicians.

If schizophrenic symptoms of the first rank are present, they are given precedence over other symptoms. If they are not, the classification tends to depend on the presence or absence of severe elevation or depression of mood, either of which may be accompanied by certain types of delusion or hallucination. In the absence of such severe affective changes, delusional experiences other than those of the first rank tend to be regarded as "paranoid," but there is disagreement as to whether these conditions should be classified with the schizophrenias or kept separate. (Nothing is lost by keeping them separate descriptively, since they can be combined, if necessary, for other purposes.) If no delusions or hallucinations are present, similiar hierarchic principles can be used to allocate the remaining conditions to a class of manic, depressive, obsessional, or anxiety disorders.

One of the principles of classification must be concerned with the problem of reactivity between syndromes. Depression may be the result of prolonged phobic anxiety. Conversely, anxiety may be induced by the experiences of depression.

In the International Pilot Study of Schizophrenia (41), it was found that clinical diagnoses of "functional" disorders could be matched fairly closely by using the set of such rules incorporated in the CATEGO program, although no single set of rules was adequate to cover the clinical practice of all the centres involved.

The problem of a cut-off or threshold point, below which no clinical classification can be made because too little information is available about key symptoms and syndromes, arose in only 2% of the series of 1202 cases collected in the International Pilot Study of Schizophrenia (41). This was because most of the cases were clinically severe. A larger proportion (10.3%), all with one or two delusional symptoms, was classified by the CATEGO program as "uncertain," but in this group a tentative classification could be made. About half of each of these kinds of uncertainty was resolved by the addition of information from the clinical history, using the Syndrome Check List. The procedure was surprisingly reliable (49). Most of the remaining uncertain cases were as difficult for clinicians to diagnose as for the CATEGO program to classify. Further development of this technique, in order to date and describe earlier episodes, would be very useful.

One further technique, the Aetiology Schedule, has also proved its usefulness. This schedule allows the specification of various organic, psychological and social factors thought to be important in aetiology. The clinician has to make a judgement as to which factors are present and how far each one contributes to the diagnosis. The contribution to standardisation is limited to the elimination of variation in coding, but this is one of the chief sources of difference between clinicians. A study of patients admitted to a hospital in Munich, using the PSE, CATEGO, the Syndrome Check List, and the Aetiology Schedule, demonstrated a very high degree of agreement between the standardised classification and clinical diagnosis, not only among the functional psychoses and neuroses, but including the alcohol, drug and personality disorders as well (52). The use of the same combination of techniques to classify disorders in a non-referred series is described by Schulsinger (34).

No statistical technique, such as cluster analysis, has been able to mimic clinical diagnosis to this degree. Of course, it may be that statistical techniques can produce new groupings, different from those already familiar to psychiatrists, but, as was suggested at the beginning of this paper, techniques of classifications are not likely to be useful unless put forward as a method of testing theory. Statistical clusters are not usually derived from any such purpose, nor are they usually subjected to the tests that clinical groupings are constantly having to undergo.

In the rest of this paper, I shall be concerned not with successes in achieving standardisation but with some of the problems that have emerged from earlier and current studies which might benefit from a good deal more attention of a similar kind. The first set of problems arises from studies of the functional psychoses, the second from studies of the "minor neuroses."

The Functional Psychoses

Perhaps the best known of the outstanding problems of classification of the functional psychoses is that of the broad versus the narrow definition of schizophrenia. Both in the US-UK Diagnostic Project (11) and in the International Pilot Study of Schizophrenia (41), it was found that there is general agreement among psychiatrists concerning a large central group of syndromes— (NS) and (AH)—which, in the absence of a cerebral pathology or a specific intoxicant such as amphetamine or alcohol, is called "schizophrenic." There was very good agreement on this. Syndromes (NS) and (AH) are combined to form the main criteria for CATEGO class S, which was present in 62% of all patients in the IPSS series who were given a clinical diagnosis of schizophrenia or paranoid psychosis.

This central core of agreement was found in all nine centres, chosen for their cultural diversity, variation in language structure, and because they represented various schools of psychiatric thought. It is important to emphasize that, although the central symptoms were highly discriminatory for a diagnosis of schizophrenia, they tended to be accompanied by many others, including other types of delusions, manic symptoms and depressive symptoms. The CATEGO program also gives rise to a class P, which consists of cases with non-nuclear delusional syndromes of various types, without predominantly manic or psychotic symptoms, and a class O, which includes purely catatonic and residual or borderline syndromes. These two classes together accounted for 20% of what was called "schizophrenic or paranoid psychosis" in the IPSS. With class S added, this makes 82%. Examination of the narrative histories and the symptoms recorded in the present state examinations of patients in classes P and O strongly suggested that many different types of psychosis were represented. In about one-third of the cases in these two classes, the categorisation was very uncertain and might rest solely on a single dubious delusional symptom or on a rating of evasiveness concerning delusions.

In one IPSS centre (Taipei) there was good agreement between a clinical diagnosis of paranoid psychosis [297] and categorisation in class P. This suggests that a common practice could be achieved if it were thought to be worthwhile, but it is clear that there is no consensus on the matter. Conditions in class P included cases characterised by "monosymptomatic" delusions, for example morbid jealousy, or a conviction that the patient's teeth were too protruberant, or that he gave off an unpleasant smell, or that others thought him homosexual, as well as more florid clinical pictures with widespread persecutory or religious or grandiose delusions. Similarly, within class O there were many different kinds of condition that might, or might not, be connected aetiologically or biologically or in other ways with more central schizophrenic conditions. Some might well have had a specific organic origin, such as encephalitis, some might be better classified as Asperger's syndrome, or the late manifestations of early childhood autism, and some might have been better regarded as specific sub-cultural states.

Example of Case History

One example will be given to illustrate the problems of classification raised by the IPSS. It is taken from Volume 1 of the IPSS report (41) and represents a group of conditions of acute excitement, seen particularly in centres in developing countries, that are difficult to classify using conventional clinical groupings. They tended to be given the diagnosis of "Schizophrenia, Other" [295.8] or "Not Otherwise Specified" [295.9], which was quite reasonable in the circumstances.

Diagnosis: Schizophrenia, Other [295.8] CATEGO class, P? [297.9]
Present episode: "The patient was perfectly well and doing his
work well some six months back, when he developed fever. It was
of low grade continuous type. He suffered from fever along with
mild headache for two days. Exact nature of the fever not known.
As soon as the fever subsided he started complaining of pain in the
gums of the molar region and so he was shown to a village doctor
who gave him some indigenous medicine to apply over his gums. He
came home and applied the medicine in the morning and, as ad-
vised, lay down on the bed. Some 1½ hours later he suddenly got
up from the bed and started abusing family members. He also
accused his father of doing wrong things and earning money by
unfair means. That day he did not take his lunch. He showed
temper episodically that day and every now and then abused his
relatives, tore his clothes and became naked; he also started getting
violent and tried to run away from the house. Hence his relatives
locked him in the room. On the following night he did not sleep
normally. He repeatedly woke up and disturbed others, saying to
them that somebody has come to the house and is knocking on the
door, why do not they open the door, although there was nothing
of that sort. He did not take a bath next day, nor did he go to
the field or take care of his cattle. All throughout the day he was
noisy and boisterous, ordering people to do this and that. He did
not talk with his wife or children. He was restless and tried to run
away from the house and so he was chained and put to bed. Suddenly on the fourth day morning he started behaving normally, took
his bath and meals, and went to the field for work. On the farm
he worked satisfactorily for the whole day. On being asked why
he was behaving like a madman, he said that he did not remember
anything. He remained apparently normal for about 8-10 days and
then again started to become violent, assaultive and restless, and
stopped going to work. He talked much and irrelevantly. He became
abusive and started interfering with others. He lost his sleep and
slept scarcely 2-3 hours at night. (Normally he sleep for 6-7 hours.)
He became irregular in taking meals. At times he took a heavy diet
and at others refused outright to take anything. He also said that
he had become very weak and from now onwards he would take
milk and butter only. This state remained for about a fortnight.
Again without any treatment he became apparently well and started
working and talking normally. He regained his sleep and appetite
and stopped showing any fads about food. He remained well for
about a fortnight and again started showing the above mentioned
symptoms. In this manner he continued behaving abnormally off
and on. He started showing these symptoms to a very severe degree
about 1½ months back. He was violent and assaultive, talking irrelevantly and much, complaining that dead people (his relatives) were
reborn and were coming to him talking with him; he often would

say to his parents and relatives, 'Look, so-and-so dead man has come to life and is talking with me.' When his relatives denied seeing any such man in the house, he would become irritable and say that they were deceiving him, they are seeing that man but want to confuse him and drive him mad. Repeatedly he used to complain of seeing dead people. He also stopped going to work, lost interest in the household work and the care of cattle which he has at home. He slept 2-3 hours and frequently disturbed his relatives in the night while they were sleeping. He often went naked and tore his clothes, without having any regard of modesty before elders and respected ones. With this complaint he was brought to the doctor."

This patient did not have any of the usual varieties of schizophrenia. He did not have mania, typical examples of which were recorded in all centres. The condition began with a fever but there were no localising features, and no organic disease was diagnosed. One of the functions of cross-cultural studies is to describe conditions of this kind, which cannot readily be accommodated within any of the theories put forward for more conventional disorders.

Before we consider the value of standardised techniques of description and classification for promoting theory-testing, it is necessary to discuss some components of morbidity other than the symptom commonly occurring in the acute functional psychiatric disorders, that we have so far been concerned with. Whatever the theory of schizophrenia, for example, it is common ground that the acute central syndromes are frequently preceded, accompanied or followed by other clinical phenomena. Two main groups of chronic symptoms are involved. The first is the well-known group of chronic "negative" symptoms, including flatness of affect, poverty of speech, slowness, underactivity, social withdrawal, and lack of motivation. These traits are highly intercorrelated and can be readily measured, in long-stay patients, by means of behaviour scales (48). Together they constitute a useful measure of the severity of one kind of chronic impairment. The social withdrawal score is highly correlated with work output at simple industrial tasks, and also with measures of central and peripheral arousal (10, 38, 48). It also represents quantitatively the individual's ability to communicate using verbal and nonverbal skills. The most severely impaired person conveys little information through his use of facial expression, voice modulation, or bodily posture, gait or gesture. In addition to these chronic negative symptoms, there may be incoherence of speech, unpredictability of associations, and a hypothesized disorder of thought.

These chronic impairments are not best measured during a "present state" examination, since they are manifested over longer periods of time and are more often observable in behavior than described by the patient. In schizophrenia, it is accepted that such impairments may be manifested during childhood (40), long before the more florid symptoms are seen.

Two other kinds of long-standing difficulty also need to be taken into account. All severe or chronic impairment is likely to be accompanied by changes in the handicapped person's self-attitudes. For example, the reaction of schizophrenic patients to a long stay in an institution has been analysed in some detail (48). The longer the stay, the more likely is the patient to lose any ability or any wish to leave, and this fact lies at the heart of institutionalism, a characteristic "secondary" handicap. Equivalent problems are likely to be encountered at home, at work, and in other facets of everyday life, and each individual has to arrive at his or her own adjustment to them.

The third kind of disadvantage is called "extrinsic" because it is handicapping even if the individual has not been ill. Someone who has had little education, who has few social or occupational skills or potentialities, or who has no family supports might well be regarded as handicapped even if he never became ill. All three types of disadvantage interact to produce the social disablement uniquely present in any given individual. The standards adopted to define disablement will, of course, vary from one social group to another (42, 46).

We may now return to the question of the definition and subclassification of "schizophrenia." We have seen that there is agreement among psychiatrists all over the world on the diagnosis of a substantial central group of conditions, defined on the basis of highly discriminating symptoms. Outside these limits, however, there is some disagreement as to which conditions should be regarded as schizophrenic. Some psychiatrists, for example, make a diagnosis purely on the basis of affective or behavioural abnormalities, particularly the chronic negative impairments and "thought disorder" even when the more characteristic syndromes are absent and there is no evidence that they have ever occurred. These chronic impairments are quite difficult to recognise reliably unless very severe, and they may have multiple causes.

On the whole, a wider range of conditions (other than those characterised by the central syndromes) tends to be included under the label "schizophrenia" in some parts of the United States and the Soviet Union than elsewhere (11, 41). Two quite different theoretical formulations are often put forward to support a broad concept of schizophrenia. One is the psychoanalytic, postulating that persisting infantile modes of thinking constitute the fundamental disorder, and that these can be recognised by experts even in the absence of more florid manifestations. The other is the multiple gene theory, which postulates a continuum between the most severe and obvious central type of schizophrenia and relatively mild, even positive and creative, traits in relatives and the general population. It will be difficult to test either kind of theory very stringently unless the symptoms that are regarded as descriptive of the more peripheral types of "schizophrenia" can be specified in such a way that psychiatrists all over the world can recognise them reliably. Work on "borderline syndromes" shows that it is possible to make some progress in this direction (19).

In due course, a multiaxial classification is required, each component of which can be specified with sufficient precision to allow reliable measurement. It will then be possible to compare series of patients diagnosed as schizophrenic, wherever the diagnosis is made and whatever the theoretical background of the psychiatrist. We have made some progress in this direction, particularly so far as the central and the paranoid syndromes are concerned, but there is still a long way to go.

A multiaxial system, in which acute symptoms, chronic impairments, secondary handicaps, and extrinsic disadvantages were all classified separately would also facilitate the comparison of course and outcome under different social conditions. Murphy and Raman (28) found that the course of "schizophrenia" was more benign in Mauritius than had been found in a follow-up study of English patients (6). A similar result has been found in the follow-up of patients in the IPSS series. Those living in developing countries seem to have a less severe course than those in more industrialised countries (31). But the "course" includes all the components of disablement mentioned earlier and it would be very helpful to be able to measure each separately, with a fair degree of reliability and precision, so that various explanations for the different results could be rigorously tested. These explanations would include one possibility that selective factors were responsible (i.e., that the conditions called "schizophrenic" were not actually comparable), and another that varying social factors were important (4, 5, 39, 48).

The practical issues are as important as the theoretical, particularly if someone who is regarded as "schizophrenic" on the basis of broad criteria, in the absence of any of the generally accepted central symptoms, is treated as though he or she did indeed have the more restricted condition. There is no evidence, for example, that the phenothiazine drugs are useful for "simple" or "sluggish" schizophrenia, if no florid symptoms are present. Questions of responsibility are also raised. A great deal then depends on local cultural, social and political factors (1, 15, 25, 27, 45), as well as on the type of theory that is adopted as a basis for the broad concept.

The Minor Neuroses

So far, we have been considering the description and classification of acute functional psychiatric disorders. In two large international studies it has proved possible to distinguish three clinical groups—schizophrenic and paranoid disorders, manic disorders, and depressive disorders—by the use of standardised techniques based on the PSE. Most of the patients examined during the course of these studies had recently been admitted to hospital and were still in the acute stage of an episode. The disorders were usually severe, therefore, and this made the application of a standard classification technique easier. The CATEGO program incorporates a set of rules that, when applied to a given profile of PSE symptoms, results in a classification into one, and only one, of 50 subclasses. These can be collapsed into a small number of classes, each of which, under specified circumstances, is equivalent to a diagnostic grouping. The program incorporates two main threshold points for the recognition of psychiatric disorders. One subclass simply contains all those who have no PSE symptoms at all. A second picks out those who have only non-specific symptoms, such as worrying, muscular tension, tiredness, poor concentration or difficulty in getting off to sleep, which do not, in themselves, suggest any particular clinical grouping. Only 2% of the 1202 cases in the IPSS did not come above these threshold points.

However, even the application of the upper of these two thresholds results in over-inclusion. Anyone with a rating of moderate depressed mood, for example, would be classified by the program as having a "depressive disorder," even if no other symptoms were present at all. Such cases rarely arose in the inpatient series, since nearly all were clinically severe.

This would not necessarily be the case in a population survey. Less than one percent of the population of countries with well-developed health services are referred for specialist advice or treatment (2, 50, 53), whereas surveys of general practice suggest that 10-15 percent of those who visit their family doctor during the course of a year are suffering from conditions that can be diagnosed as psychiatric (35). Population surveys have suggested even higher proportions of undiagnosed "cases" (36).

Earlier epidemiologists dealt with the problem of comparability by trying to use the same diagnostic criteria, whether they were examining clinic patients or a sample of people drawn from the general population. Which factors were taken into account and what loadings were allocated in each case were matters for private but presumably consistent judgement. The disadvantage was that the decision in each case was necessarily unique and unspecifiable in precise terms; the same process of decision-making could not be matched by other workers.

Another way to approach the problem is to set diagnosis aside altogether and to use instead an estimate of "significant" psychiatric disorder based, for example, on a threshold score from a symptom check-list (18), or a global judgement agreed by several workers (7, 8). Considerable methodological advance has been achieved by improving the reproducibility and repeatability of such procedures, but the problem of exact specification of the threshold points, as well as the reliable classification of the "cases" so found, has not been solved.

One of the central components of the problem is that of the threshold level below which it is difficult to recognise, within a set of symptoms elicited by a standard procedure, any pattern that clearly falls into one of the major ICD categories of functional psychosis or neurosis. It is fair to say that no epidemiological study so far published has attempted to define this threshold in terms that could be replicated from one project to another. The problems involved can be illustrated by reference to the depressive disorders. The minimum criterion, of course, is the presence of depressed mood but, by itself, this is quite common, and few psychiatrists would wish to make a diagnosis of depressive disorder, still less to initiate biological or psychological treatments, on this basis alone. If there are other symptoms suggestive of a depressive disorder, such as pathological guilt or psychomotor retardation, the presence of at least a "borderline disorder"* can be postulated. Criteria of this kind can be

---

* The term borderline is here used to indicate the conditions which have some but not all of the characteristics of a definite disorder. It should be distinguished from the way it is used in other papers in this symposium.

laid down fairly precisely. The presence of yet further symptoms makes the classification even more definite. The Feighner standards, for example, which require the presence of (a) depression for at least a month, (b) 5 out of 8 other symptoms and (c) the absence of other syndromes, might be taken as fairly definite criteria. All the "present state" information needed is present in the PSE (16).

It should be emphasized that procedures of this kind have a purely clinical foundation. Such a justification is based upon the experience of our teachers and upon our own clinical theories. It may be wrong. But the great advantage of laying down precise criteria is that if they are wrong they can be shown to be so. The theories are testable.

We have recently used an index of definition of psychiatric disorders in various series of southeast London, all examined using the 9th edition of the Present State Examination. In a series of recently admitted in-patients with functional disorders, 88% had conditions that could quite definitely be classified according to the criteria laid down in a computer program. Nearly all the rest had borderline disorders. In a series of out-patients, 83% had borderline or definite disorders. In a random sample of the general population in the same area, 12% had borderline or definite disorders (mostly depressive) and nearly all these were borderline (44). Only one person had symptoms that met the Feighner criteria for a depressive disorder.

This was in an inner suburb of London where the general morbidity is likely to be quite high. Rutter and his colleagues (30), for example, found twice as much psychiatric disorder among children as in a less urban area in southern England.

John Orley (personal communication) has used the same technique in two villages in Uganda, where he and a local colleague interviewed nearly every adult. Overall, 25% of the adult populations in the villages had borderline or definite conditions, i.e., twice as many as in southeast London. The frequency was much the same in men and women. When the symptom profiles of people with borderline or definite depressive disorders in the Ugandan villages were compared with the profiles of Londoners with equivalent conditions, it was found that symptoms such as guilt and subjective anergia were more common in the villages.

Obviously this kind of work needs to be repeated in many other settings, but it does look as though the technique is a useful one. We also found that non-medical interviewers could use the technique as well as psychiatrists (work to be published). Copeland et al. (12), pointed out, however, that one has to be careful about the frame of reference of the interviewer. Psychiatrists tend to have a model of disorder based upon their clinic experience, i.e., they tend to rate less disorder in a general population than non-medical interviewers, who tend to have a model of disorder based on their own personal experience and are therefore likely to rate symptoms more readily. These tendencies can be corrected by training. Non-medical interviewers, given the same training on the PSE as psychiatrists, can learn to adopt the same standards. They can then achieve a reasonable degree of reliability, judged by simultaneous ratings of one interview, or ratings of tape-recorded interviews, or by interviews repeated within a week of each other.

THEORIES ABOUT PROBLEMS AND THEORIES ABOUT DISEASES

Thus, both for the functional psychoses, and for the neuroses found in general population surveys, a good deal can be done to make the process of case-identification and classification more reliable and communicable. This means that theories about them can be more rigorously tested. But this is not everything. Patients bring problems to their doctors, multifaceted and multicausal. A man may be worried about impotence, a woman about a fear that she is not attractive to her husband. Either may complain of marital discord, or of a tendency to drink too much, or of truanting by a child, or simply of vague bodily pains. Each of these complaints will have biological, psychological and social components. Not one of these problems needs necessarily be accompanied by complaints of symptoms that can be identified as falling into any of the syndromes of functional psychosis or neurosis we have been discussing, although it would be generally agreed that any of them *could* be associated with such syndromes. In other words, the conditions that psychiatrists are asked to advise upon, and to treat if they can, cover an extremely wide spectrum, and useful disease theories can only be put forward for a relatively restricted group. Here I am reverting to the position taken in the early part of the paper.

This is not a defensive position. There is no reason why disease theories should have to be adopted when there is no evidence at all that they are useful. Doctors acquire expertise in a wide variety of techniques of helping people and they should be able to refer patients elsewhere when they know their own resources are not equal to the problem. Medicine is *not* simply a matter of treating, or advising about, diseases.

Nevertheless, disease theories and the various ways of testing them do form an essential part of the doctor's special knowledge. If he does not possess this knowledge, he is practising under false pretenses. The presence of definable psychiatric syndromes of depression, in mild form, may be purely reactive, or they may be mild forms of conditions that can be treated biologically. One of the major problems for future study concerns the elucidation of the relationship between the severe depressive disorders met among inpatients and outpatients, that frequently respond to pharmacological treatment and concerning which disease theories are confidently put forward, and the lesser depressive disorders (such as those defined as "borderline" by the index of definition) that often seem to be immediately reactive to difficulties experienced in the patient's social or psychological environment. There is a danger here of being beguiled by a purely semantic controversy between supporters of a dimensional and supporters of a categorical school of thought. Ice, water and steam are categories (although the distinctions between them are not absolute), but one underlying dimension of temperature underlies all three. We have found that total PSE score is quite a good measure of clinical severity in the lesser and depressive disorders but that, as the score increases, extra symptoms of depression become manifest—first depressed mood itself, then subjective anergia, then pathological guilt, and so on.

No one familiar with diabetes or hypertension will be disposed to argue that disease cannot have a dimensional basis. On the other hand, no one familiar with recent successful attempts at social skills training, or removing isolated specific phobias, or helping to educate severely handicapped children and adults to find ways round their disabilities will wish to say that disease theories are the be-all and the end-all of medicine. They are not. But to assume that this conclusion means that disease theories are of no value in psychiatry is to give in to the Yahoos.

Fortunately, it is not necessary to choose between one and the other. An enormous amount of sterile controversy has stemmed from protagonists taking up mutually exclusive positions. The role model of the doctor is broad. He acts, upon occasion, as a teacher, psychologist, social worker, pastoral counselor, or befriender. Any narrow view of the doctor's role, based on the sole function of biologic diagnosis, is likely to lead to a stereotyped mislabeling of the medical profession and a thorough misunderstanding of the value of diagnosis. Doctors are presented with problems that have multiple causes. Some components of these problems can most effectively be helped by applying a disease theory. Many others need other approaches. If a doctor fails to spot that he can diminish disability and distress by making and acting on the right theory, he is failing his patient. That is why it is important to take the diagnostic process seriously, and to try to make is as efficient as possible. Within a broad medical framework, the sharper our diagnostic tools, the better.

SUMMARY

Any set of techniques designed to standardise the procedures underlying clinical diagnosis can be successful only if its limitations are recognised. The advantages and disadvantages are two sides of the same coin. The main value of developing reliable techniques of describing and classifying clinical syndromes is to improve the testing of explanatory theories by improving the comparability of case-finding. This can be done with fair success within the acute and severe functional psychoses and neuroses. There is also some evidence that case-finding in general population samples can also be improved, using an extension of the same principles. Thus it is beginning to be possible to look for "cases," in non-referred samples, with a known degree of similarity to those already familiar in inpatient and outpatient series.

This process of working from the known to the unknown illuminates several areas where further work might be fruitful. Among these are: the delineation of new varieties of psychosis, particularly in certain cultural contexts; the further testing of theories based on narrow and broad concepts of schizophrenia; the subdivision of paranoid psychoses not accompanied by central schizophrenic symptoms; the elucidation of certain conditions, often called schizophrenic, although there are no central or paranoid symptoms; and the development of methods of case-finding in non-referred populations.

The measurement of chronic impairments, secondary handicaps and extrinsic disadvantages, and their contribution to social disablement, would allow even more stringent theory-testing—in particular, tests of theories concerning factors affecting the course of psychiatric disorders.

Although this paper is mainly concerned with how diagnosis can be made more reliable and communicable, it is emphasized that diagnosis is only one part of a doctor's work. The tools of diagnosis can be sharpened, but whether they are used, and if so, how, is the responsibility of the clinician. His decisions must be based on a full knowledge of all the patient's problems, and it will be very unusual for him to act upon disease theories alone.

ACKNOWLEDGEMENTS

Experience derived from the US-UK Diagnostic Project and the W.H.O. International Pilot Study of Schizophrenia, as well as from a long series of studies conducted by, or in collaboration with, the MRC Social Psychiatry Unit, has been invaluable in formulating the views expressed in this paper. Full details of those taking part in this work are given in the instruction manual (49). The more recent work, based on studies of non-referred populations, has been carried out in collaboration with Professor G. W. Brown, Dr. Scott Henderson, Dr. M. McCarthy, Dr. J. Orley and Dr. H. Schulsinger. Dr. Julian Leff and Dr. Sheila Mann have been particularly involved in developing the index of definition.

REFERENCES

1. Arens, R. *Make Mad the Guilty*. Springfield, Ill.: Thomas, 1969.
2. Bahn, A. K., Gardner, E. A., Alltop, L., Knatterud, G. L., & Solomon, M. Comparative studies of rates of admission and prevalence for psychiatric facilities in four register areas. *American Journal of Public Health*, 56, 2033, 1966.
3. Baker, J. R. *Race*. London: Oxford University Press, 1974.
4. Brown, G. W., & Birley, J. L. T. Crisis and life changes and the onset of schizophrenia. *Journal of Health and Human Behavior*, 9, 203-214, 1968.
5. Brown, G. W., Birley, J. L. T., & Wing, J. K. Influence of family life on the course of schizophrenic disorders: A replication. *British Journal of Psychiatry*, 121, 241-258, 1972.
6. Brown, G. W., Bone, M., Dalison, B., & Wing, J. K. *Schizophrenia and Social Care*. London: Oxford University Press, 1966.
7. Brown, G. W., Bhrolchain, M., & Harris, T. Social class and psychiatric disturbance among women in an urban population. *Sociology*, 9, 225-254, 1975.
8. Brown, G. W., Sklair, F., Harris, T., & Birley, J. L. T. Life events and psychiatric disorders: Some methodological issues. *Psychological Medicine*, 3, 74-87, 1973.
9. Carstairs, G. M. Cultural elements in the response to treatment. In Reuck, A. V. S., and Porter, R. (Eds.), *Transcultural Psychiatry*. London: Churchill, 1965.
10. Catterson, A., Bennett, D. H., & Freudenberg, R. K. A survey of long term schizophrenic patients. *British Journal of Psychiatry*, 109, 750, 1963.
11. Cooper, J. E., Kendell, R. E., Gurland, B. J., Sharpe, L., Copeland, J. R. M., & Simon, R. *Psychiatric Diagnosis in New York and London*. Maudsley Monograph No. 20. London: Oxford University Press, 1972.
12. Copeland, J., Kelleher, M. J., Gourlay, A. J., & Smith, A. M. R. Influence of psychiatric training, medical qualification, and paramedical training on the rating of abnormal behavior. *Psychological Medicine*, 5, 89-95, 1975.
13. Dubos, R. *Man Adapting*. New Haven: Yale University Press, 1965.
14. Ellenberger, H. F. *The Discovery of the Unconscious*. London: Allen Lane, 1970.
15. Ennis, B. *Prisoners of Psychiatry: Mental Patients, Psychiatrists and the Law*. New York: Harcourt Brace Jovanovich, 1972.

16. Feighner, J. P., Robins, E., Guze, S. B., Woodruff, R. A., Winokur, G., & Munoz, R. Diagnostic criteria for use in psychiatric research. *Archives of General Psychiatry*, 26, 57-63, 1972.
17. Foulds, G. A., & Bedford, A. Hierarchy of classes of personal illness. *Psychological Medicine*, 5, 181-192, 1975.
18. Goldberg, D. *The Detection of Psychiatric Illness by Questionnaire.* London: Oxford University Press, 1972.
19. Grinker, R., Werble, B., & Drye, R. C. *The Borderline Syndrome.* New York: Basic Books, 1966.
20. Haslam, J. *Observations on Madness and Melancholy.* London: Hayden, 1809.
21. Hempel, C. G. Introduction to problems of taxonomy. In Zubin, J. (Ed.), *Field Studies in the Mental Disorders.* New York: Grune and Stratton, 1959.
22. Hirsch, S. R., & Leff, J. P. *Abnormality in Parents of Schizophrenics: A Review of the Literature and an Investigation of Communication Defects and Deviances.* London: Oxford University Press, 1975.
23. Itard, J. M. G. (1801, 1807). *The Wild Boy of Aveyron.* English translation by G. and M. Humphrey, 1932. New York: Appleton-Century-Crofts, 1962.
24. Kanner, L. Autistic disturbances of affective contact. *Nerv. Child*, 2, 217, 1943.
25. Khodorovich, T. *The Case of Leonid Plyushch.* London: Hurst, 1976.
26. McKeown, T., et al. *Medical History and Medical Care.* London: Oxford University Press, 1971.
27. Morosov, G. Letter in reply to Wing. *British Medical Journal*, 3, 40, 1974.
28. Murphy, H. B. M., & Raman, A. C. The chronicity of schizophrenia in indigenous tropical peoples: Results of a 12 year follow-up survey. *British Journal of Psychiatry*, 118, 489-497, 1971.
29. Pledge, H. T. *Science Since 1500.* London: H.M.S.O., 1939.
30. Rutter, M. Why are London children so disturbed? *Proceedings of the Royal Society of Medicine*, 66, 1221-1225, 1973.
31. Sartorius, N., Jablensky, A., & Strömgren, E. Second Rochester International Conference on Schizophrenia. To be published, 1977.
32. Scharfetter,, C., Moerbt, H., & Wing, J. K. Diagnosis of functional psychoses: Comparison of clinical and computerized classifications. *Arch. Psychiat. Nervenkr.*, 222, 61-67, 1976.
33. Schneider, K. *Clinical Psychopathology*, 5th edition. Trans: Hamilton, M. W. New York: Grune and Stratton, 1959.
34. Schulsinger, H. A ten-year follow-up of children of schizophrenic mothers. *Acta Psychiatrica Scandinavica*, 53, 371-386, 1976.
35. Shepherd, M., Cooper, B., Brown, A. C., & Kalton, G. W. *Psychiatric Illness in General Practice.* London: Oxford University Press, 1966.
36. Srole, L., Langner, T. S., Michael, S. T., Opler, M. K., & Rennie, T. A. *Mental Health in the Metropolis: The Midtown Manhattan Study.* New York: McGraw-Hill, 1962.
37. Szasz, T. Schizophrenia: The sacred symbol of psychiatry. *British Journal of Psychiatry*, 129, 308-316, 1976.
38. Venables, P., & Wing, J. K. Level of arousal and the subclassification of schizophrenia. *Archives of General Psychiatry*, 1, 114-119, 1962.
39. Vaughn, C. E., & Leff, J. P. The influence of family and social factors on the course of psychiatric illness. *British Journal of Psychiatry*, 129, 125-137, 1976.
40. Watt, N. F., & Lubensky, A. W. Childhood roots of schizophrenia. *Journal of Consulting and Clinical Psychology*, 44, 363-375, 1976.
41. World Health Organisation. *The International Pilot Study of Schizophrenia.* Geneva: W.H.O., 1973.

42. Wing, J. K. Impairments in schizophrenia: A rational basis for social treatment. In Wirt, R. D., Winokur, G., and Roff, M. (Eds.), *Life History Research in Psychopathology*, Vol. 4. Minneapolis: University of Minnesota Press, 1975.
43. Wing, J. K. (Ed.). Classification of psychiatric disorders. *Psychiatric Annals*, Vols. 6 and 7. 1976a.
44. Wing, J. K. A technique for comparing psychiatric morbidity in inpatient and outpatient series with that found in general population samples. *Psychological Medicine*, 6, 665-671, 1976b.
45. Wing, J. K. *Reasoning about Madness*. London and New York: Oxford University Press, 1977a.
46. Wing, J. K. Social influences on the course of schizophrenia. Second Rochester International Conference on Schizophrenia. (To be published). 1977b.
47. Wing, J. K., Bennett, D. H., & Denham, J. *The Industrial Rehabilitation of Long-Stay Schizophrenic Patients*. Med. Res. Council memo. No. 42. London: H. M. S. O., 1964.
48. Wing, J. K., & Brown, G. W. *Institutionalism and Schizophrenia*. London: Cambridge University Press, 1970.
49. Wing, J. K., Cooper, J. E., & Sartorius, N. *The Description and Classification of Psychiatric Symptoms: An Instruction Manual for the PSE and CATEGO System*. London: Cambridge University Press, 1974.
50. Wing, J. K., & Hailey, A. M. (Eds.). *Evaluating a Community Psychiatric Service: The Camberwell Register, 1964-1971*. London: Oxford University Press, 1972.
51. Wing, J. K., & Nixon, J. Discriminating symptoms in schizophrenia. *Archives of General Psychiatry*. 32, 853-859, 1975.
52. Wing, J. K., Nixon, J., Von Cranach, M., & Strauss, A. Further developments of the PSE and CATEGO system. Accepted for publication: W.H.O., 1977.
53. Wing, L., Wing, J. K., Hailey, A. M., Bahn, A. K., Smith, H. E., & Baldwin, J. A. The use of psychiatric services in three urban areas: An international case register study. *Sociological Psychiatry*, 2, 158-167, 1967.
54. Wynne, L. C. Methodologic and conceptual issues in the study of schizophrenics and their families. In Rosenthal, D., and Kety, S. S. (Eds.), *The Transmission of Schizophrenia*. London and New York: Pergamon, 1968.
55. Wynne, L. C. Family research on the pathogenesis of schizophrenia. In Doncet, P., and Laurin, C. (Eds.), *Problems of Psychosis*. Excerpta Medica International Congress Series, No. 194, 1971.

6

The Scope and Validity of the Schizophrenic Spectrum Concept

PAUL H. WENDER, M.D.

It is the purpose of this paper to discuss the contributions of the adoption studies of schizophrenia to our understanding of the nature and extent of the schizophrenia spectrum concept. Most people acquainted with the adoption studies of schizophrenia realize that they have helped distinguish the respective roles of nature and nurture in the etiology of these disorders. What many people have not reflected on is that they also have helped us to document the existence of and define the phenomenology of the "schizophrenic spectrum." In fact, at present they provide the only logical method for characterizing the schizophrenic spectrum and defining its limits.

It is usual, when presenting scientific results, to do so in the manner of the Euclidian theorem. The authors begin by stating their hypotheses and their implications, continue with the experiments they performed and the data obtained, and finish with the conclusions which inevitably follow from the data and which are directly relevant to the hypotheses. Anyone who has conducted scientific experiments realizes that this method of reporting is an artificial convention which bears no relationship to what scientists actually do. They may sometimes start at the beginning, but often they start in the middle; in either event, only if

Research reported in this paper was supported in part by NIMH Grant MH 255 15.

they are lucky do they reach a meaningful end. I mention this well known, but infrequently acknowledged phenomenon, because what took place in the adoption studies of the schizophrenias was not a neat postulation of the existence of a schizophrenic spectrum followed by the documentation of its existence. What happened is that we began by considering its possible existence and pulled ourselves up by our logical bootstraps. It will be useful, therefore, to document what we did and how the relevant information followed from our actions.

When we began the adoption studies, we were handicapped by an obvious theoretical impasse. We wished to study the contributions of nature and nurture to the etiology of the schizophrenias, but we were unsure what conditions the schizophrenias comprised. We decided to resolve the issue empirically by studying a group of conditions to which the term "schizophrenia" had been applied without knowing whether or not that application was valid. By the designs of the studies, which I shall discuss, we hoped not only to determine the contributions of nature and nurture to the etiology of these disorders, but to determine whether these disorders could be meaningfully grouped together.

The term "schizophrenia" has been variously used historically to refer to a wide variety of psychiatric disorders. Historically, as is well known, Kraepelin proposed that certain seemingly different psychoses (hebephrenia, catatonia, and certain paranoid states) could be grouped together and separated from other psychoses. He designated this group as "dementia praecox," an illness characterized by early onset, progressive course, and flagrant psychiatric symptomatology. Bleuler further elaborated on Kraepelin's subgrouping, vastly broadening the category to include less severely ill individuals, and renamed the syndrome as the "group of schizophrenias." Bleuler asserted that all the affected individuals had, despite their seeming behavioral heterogeneity, certain "primary" (basic) psychological abnormalities which they held in common. These included: cognitive impairments not related to intelligence and manifested as "thought disorder"; abnormalities of emotional reactivity which included unresponsiveness, marked ambivalence and alterations in relation to other people; and finally a predilection for withdrawal into fantasy. These constituted defining attributes of the syndrome. This group of individuals was, Bleuler felt, also likely to develop more obvious "secondary" symptoms, not necessarily present or essential for the diagnosis, included psychological manifestations such as abnormal perceptual phenomena (illusions and hallucinations), elaborate intellectual misconceptions (delu-

sions), and aberrant motor behavior (catatonia). Bleuler's definition was far more encompassing than Kraepelin's: Bleuler used the term "schizophrenia" to refer to all individuals with "primary symptoms" while Kraepelin's "dementia praecox" referred to those individuals who manifested both the primary and secondary symptomatology of Bleuler. I have offered this brief historical digression to highlight one source of the ambiguity regarding the meaning of the term "schizophrenia." In European psychiatry, it is generally used in a narrow sense to refer to Kraepelin's "dementia praecox"; in the United States, the term is applied in Bleuler's sense and, ipso facto, includes a much broader range of psychopathology. In the United States the term "schizophrenia" is variously used to refer to: chronic schizophrenia; acute reactive schizophrenia; borderline schizophrenia; and schizoid states.

Not fully knowing what we wished to investigate and not wishing to prematurely foreclose the issue, we decided to investigate these four major forms of psychiatric illness variously designated as "schizophrenic" in current American psychiatry. For our studies we have defined them as described below.

The first illness corresponds to Kraepelin's dementia praecox and is variously termed "process," chronic, or "true" schizophrenia. Individuals with this illness are characterized by a history of poor pre-psychotic adjustment, having tended to have been introverted and "shut-in"; they have had few peer contacts and few heterosexual relationships; they frequently remained unmarried, the males particularly, and have shown poor occupational adjustment. The onset of the illness tends to be gradual and without any clear-cut psychological precipitants. The illness itself is characterized by conspicuous manifestations of "primary" Bleulerian characteristics; the "secondary" characteristics (hallucinations, delusions, etc.) are often present as well. The illness does not tend to respond well to treatment and its course tends to be chronic.

The second form of illness, designated "reactive schizophrenia" or "acute schizophrenic reaction" in the United States, presents an appreciably different clinical picture. Individuals suffering from this disorder have generally manifested a relatively good premorbid personality adjustment in terms of their interpersonal relationships, heterosexual adjustment, and work history. The illness tends to have a relatively rapid onset and may have appeared in the context of psychological precipitants. The presenting picture is characterized by: the clear-cut presence of secondary symptoms and comparatively lesser evidence of primary ones; the presence of depressive or manic affect (so that the illness may be designated as schizoaffective); and a cloudy rather than a clear sensorium. The illness itself tends to respond to phenothiazines and electroshock therapy. The long-term prognosis is fairly good, although a certain fraction of acute schizophrenias eventually goes on to develop chronic schizophrenic states. European psychiatrists do not consider acute schizophrenic reactions to be related to the schizophrenias, as is indicated by their designation of the syndrome as "schizophreniform psychosis" or "psychogenic psychosis."

A third group of illnesses which are considered in the United States to be related to the schizophrenias are those designated by a number of terms including "pseudo-neurotic schizophrenia," "borderline schizophrenia," and "ambulatory schizophrenia" (to present only a few of a host of synonyms). The descriptions of this group of disorders vary considerably. Several authors have proposed that a variety of syndromes be designated as "borderline," basing their groupings on criteria ranging from phenomenology to inferences regarding intrapsychic constructs. For our initial purposes, we decided to define this category as referring to individuals manifesting the types and degree of psychopathology described by Hoch and Polatin (1) in their discussion of "pseudoneurotic schizophrenia." This category would therefore include individuals having a chronic history of psychological maladaptation with abnormalities in the following areas: 1) *Thinking*—strange, vague, illogical mentation which tends to ignore reality, logic and experience, and results in poor adaptation to life experiences; 2) *Affective life*—characterized by "anhedonia," the inability to experience intense pleasure, so that the individuals report a history of never having been happy (although they may never have been seriously depressed); 3) *Interpersonal relations*—characterized by a tendency to polar opposites which may include either the absence of deep, intense involvement with other people or excessively "deep" and dependent involvement with others. There also exist possible difficulties in sexual adjustment which may be characterized by either a very low sexual drive or a promiscuous and chaotic pattern of sexual interaction; 4) *Psychopathology*—characterized not only by its intensity but by its lack of constancy with multiple neurotic manifestations that may shift frequently (obsessive concerns, phobias, conversion symptoms, psychosomatic symptoms, etc.); severe, widespread anxiety and occasionally short-lived episodes, designated as "micropsychotic," during which the individual experiences transient delusions, hallucinations, feelings of depersonalization or de-realization. The course of these disturbances tends to be lifelong, generally without deterioration, and the illnesses seem refractory to neuroleptic drugs.

The fourth group of illnesses are symptomatically the most distant from and share the fewest characteristics with chronic schizophrenia. Individuals with this disorder were designated by Kretschmer (3) as "schizothymes" and by Kallman (2) as "schizoidia"; in the United States they are usually referred to as "schizoid." The attributes of individuals in this category have been variously described. The scope of Kretchmer's term may be seen in this description of the relatives of a chronic schizophrenic, all of whom manifest the basic trait, "schizothymia." The patient in question had three brothers: one was shy, conscientious, competent; another was quiet, serious, logical and sociable and desired "to get away"; the third was an inventor who was described as stormy and depressed, passionate, restless, with an equally strong desire to "get away." The patient's mother had had a short period of paranoia when she had been alcoholic; she was described as sensitive, humorless, pedantic, depressed and affected with the repetitive family desire to "get away." The patient's father was chronically paranoid, eccentric, misanthropic, and depressed. Which of these attributes constitutes the essential manifestation of the trait is unclear; the cluster appears to be more important than the individual characteristics and there is no characteristic whose presence appears to be necessary for the diagnosis. Similar attributes—and the same problems in defining the essential symptoms—are found in Kallman's descriptions. His schizophrenia-like personalities, individuals having "schizoidia," are characterized as either: "abnormal types . . . with schizophrenic deficits following an . . . unusually mild or hidden psychotic episode . . . (or showing) autistic introversion, emotional inadequacy, sudden surges of temperament and inappropriate motor responses to emotional stimuli and in whom such symptoms . . . as bigotry, pietism, avarice, superstition, obstinacy or crankiness" strongly color the personality.

As may be seen, the clarity and specificity of the syndromes decrease as we move from the chronic schizophrenias to the schizoid states. Nonetheless, we felt their usefulness would be an empirical question. We would determine if we could reliably agree upon these diagnoses and, if we could, we would see if they clustered together genetically, suggesting an interrelationship between them.

Indeed, the studies conducted do suggest a genetic relationship between these four disorders. How they do so is best explained by a fairly detailed description of the studies. First, let me discuss their rationale.

All stem from the repeated observation, accepted both by psychodynamicists and psychiatric geneticists, that schizophrenia clusters in families. The two groups explain this observation in two different ways. One school states that the clustering of schizophrenia occurs because of psychosocial transmission, that individuals exposed to the same psychological environment will manifest similar behaviors and/or psychopathology. The other school argues that the clustering occurs because members of the same family share the same genes. In most instances the issue cannot be resolved logically since family members share both genes and environment with the schizophrenic patient. The strategy of studying adopted persons avoids this problem since those sharing genes with the patient and those sharing an environment with him are different people.

In the first group of studies, the Family Studies (4, 5), we elected to investigate the prevalence and nature of psychopathology among the biological and adopted relatives of a group of adopted schizophrenics, the Index Group, and a group of adopted non-schizophrenic individuals, the Control Group. The major focus of the study was to determine the relative contributions of genetic and experiential factors in the genesis of schizophrenia, but, as will be seen, the data obtained also shed light on the relationship between the four putative illnesses in the schizophrenic spectrum. The logic of the Family Studies was that if there were genetic contributions to the etiology of the schizophrenias, we should find increased psychopathology among the biological relatives of the adopted schizophrenics, the Index Group, as compared to Controls, even though the Index Group had had no personal contact with these biological relatives. Contrariwise, if experiential factors played a role in the genesis of schizophrenia, we would anticipate finding increased schizophrenia or schizophrenia-like psychopathology among the members of the adoptive family with whom the adopted schizophrenics, as compared to the adoptive families of the Controls, were raised.

We began by locating a population of approximately 5,500 adult adoptees. By cross-indexing them with a central registry of hospitalization for mental illnesses, we determined which of these adoptees had been diagnosed as definitely or possibly "schizophrenic." Reviewing the records ourselves, we decided that 17 adoptees could be diagnosed as chronic schizophrenics, 7 as acute schizophrenics, and 9 as borderline schizophrenics. For each of these subjects an adopted control was selected from the records of non-psychiatrically diagnosed adoptees. Each of these control subjects matched the schizophrenic index case very closely in terms of age, sex, duration of stay with biological parents, and the socioeconomic class of the adoptive parents with whom each was placed. By means of other registries, we identified the biological and adoptive parents, siblings, and half-siblings of the Index cases and Controls. Each of these relatives was then diagnosed by two techniques: first, by cross-indexing their names with the central registry of mental illness, obtaining the records, and blindly diagnosing the cases; and, second, by direct interview, obtained blindly and followed by a blind clinical evaluation of the records. We were able to obtain a detailed psychiatric interview on 90% of the relatives who had not died or emigrated, and partial information on an additional 4%. In the data analysis, only the interview data will be presented. Having diagnosed the case material, we then inspected the distribution of psychopathology among the four classes of relatives. The summary of the findings is presented in Table I.

What may be seen from an overall inspection of the data is that there is an increase of certain and uncertain schizophrenic psychopathology only among the biological relatives of the Index Group, a finding compatible with a genetic mechanism of transmission of these disorders. There is no significant increase of schizophrenic psychopathology among the adopted relatives, a finding compatible with the hypothesis that family psychopathology does not play a necessary role in the genesis of the schizophrenic disorders.

A second question, one critical for this discussion, relates to the prevalence of schizophrenic psychopathology in the relatives of the three subgroups which form the Index Group: the chronic schizophrenics (S_1), the acute schizophrenics (S_2), and the borderline schizophrenics (S_3). Each of these subgroups may be considered to be a member of the schizophrenic spectrum if, and only if, increased definite schizophrenic psychopathology is found among the relatives of individuals in the subgroup.

Before discussing this data, we must digress for a moment and deal with what happened as a result of interviewing all the available relatives of the subjects and the subjects themselves. As may be remembered, we selected the Control Adoptees only on the basis of their never having received an official psychiatric diagnosis. Obviously, this constitutes a very weak index of psychopathology. When the subjects, including the Controls, were interviewed, it was found that some of the Controls had emigrated or were dead and could therefore not be interviewed, that some manifested schizophrenic or schizophrenic-like psychopathology, and that some had other psychiatric diagnoses. Since our comparison de-

Table I

Schizophrenia Spectrum

Type of Relatives	Number Identified	Number Interviewed	Total in Schizophrenia Spectrum N %^d	Definite (S)			Uncertain D	Total S & D	Schizoid Inadequate Personality
				Chronic S1 N %	Latent S3 N %	Total S1 & S3 N %	D1,D2D3 N %	N %	N %
Biological Index	173	118	37 (21.9)	5 (2.9)	6 (3.5)	11 (6.4)	13 (7.5)	24 (13.9)	13 (7.5)
All biological controls	174	140	19 (10.9)	0 (0)	3 (1.7)	3 (1.7)	3 (1.7)	6 (3.4)	13 (7.5)
p (all index vs. all controls)		n.s.	0.006	0.03	0.25	0.026	0.009	0.0004	n.s.
Adoptive Index	74	35	4 (5.4)	1 (1.4)	0 (0)	1 (1.4)	1 (1.4)	2 (2.7)	2 (2.7)
All adoptive controls	91	48	7 (7.7)	1 (1.1)	1 (1.1)	2 (2.2)	3 (3.3)	5 (5.5)	2 (2.2)
p (all index vs. all controls)		n.s.	n.s.	n.s.	n.s.	n.s.	n.s.	n.s.	n.s.

pended on examining the relatives of schizophrenic and non-schizophrenic Controls, it makes sense to compare the Index Cases with the Controls who were interviewed and who possessed no schizophrenic features. There were 24 such individuals. Now, looking at the distribution of biological relatives for the schizophrenic (S_1) and borderline schizophrenic (S_3) subgroups, what do we find?

TABLE II

Borderline (S_3) or Doubtful Borderline (D_3) Schizophrenia
in the Relatives of Chronic and Borderline
Schizophrenics, Probands and Controls

Proband Diagnosis	Relatives with Information	First Diagnosis of Relative S_3 D_3	First or Second Diagnosis of Relative S_3 D_3
Chronic Schizophrenia	102	8a	16b
Borderline Schizophrenia	47	3c	5d
Acute Schizophrenia	22	4	4e
Screened Controls	112	1	1

Fisher exact probability Proband relatives vs. screened Controls relatives
  a p$<$.01
  b p$<$.001
  c p$<$.08
  d p$<$.01
  e p$<$.04

As shown in Table II, we find that of the 102 biological relatives of the chronic schizophrenics 8 had been given a first diagnosis of certain (S) or doubtful borderline schizophrenia, and that 16 had been given a first or second choice diagnosis of borderline or doubtful borderline schizophrenia. Both findings are statistically significant. Similarly, inspecting the prevalence of borderline or doubtful borderline schizophrenia among the biological relatives of the borderline schizophrenics, we find that three had received a first diagnosis of certain or probable borderline schizophrenia and that five had received a first or second choice diagnosis of borderline or doubtful borderline schizophrenia. As may be seen, the former finding approaches, while the latter attains, statistical significance.

Now, it should be noted that an inspection of the prevalence of borderline or doubtful borderline schizophrenia among the biological relatives of the adopted chronic schizophrenics tells us two things. First, it tells us that the two disorders are related and that "borderline schizophrenia" is indeed a genetic relative of chronic schizophrenia. Second, the increased prevalence of borderline schizophrenia among the biological relatives of the borderline schizophrenics tells us that this disorder "breeds true," that is, that this disorder can be transmitted genetically.

What about the acute schizophrenias? Are they related to the chronic schizophrenias? One obvious problem we face in answering this question is that our sample is small. We began with 7 acute schizophrenic cases who had 14 first-grade relatives (parents and full siblings) and 18 second-degree relatives (half-siblings). If genetic factors play a role in the etiology of the acute schizophrenias, how many relatives with what kind of illnesses should we anticipate finding among the biological relatives of the 7 acute schizophrenics? A study conducted by McCabe and Strömgren (6) provides us with some base-rate data. Their findings suggest that the risk for reactive psychosis (a condition which appears to be related to what we designate as acute schizophrenia) is approximately 7% among the full siblings of reactive psychotics. In this study we found no acute schizophrenic reactions, certain or doubtful, among the biological relatives of the acute schizophrenics.

Does this mean that this disorder does not have genetic contributants? If the true risk figure is indeed 7%, we would anticipate that 1 to 2 biological relatives (depending on whether the number of half-siblings is divided by two) would be anticipated to develop acute schizophrenic reactions. Unfortunately, for a population of this small size, one standard deviation is approximately 5% or 1 to 2 persons. In other words, given this small population, we cannot determine if our finding of no acute schizophrenia among the biological relatives is significantly different from chance expectation.

But we have not exhausted our analysis of this case material. Strömgren also reports an approximate prevalence of 8% for "constitutional psychopathy" and "neurosis" among the siblings of reactive psychotics. Now it is hard to know exactly what is meant by "constitutional psychopathy" and "neurosis," but it is tenable that these terms refer to a group of individuals akin to those we designated as "doubtful schizophrenics." Since doubtful schizophrenia has been shown to be increased among the relatives of chronic or borderline schizophrenics, the finding that doubtful schizophrenia was increased among the relatives of acute schizophrenics would *suggest* that the acute schizophrenics were related to the chronic and borderline schizophrenics. It is therefore of interest to examine the prevalence of doubtful schizophrenia among the relatives of our acute schizophrenics as compared to the relatives of the chronic and borderline schizophrenics and the controls. Depending on whether one employs conservative measures or not, the prevalence of doubtful schizophrenia is found to be between 13 and 18% among the biological relatives of the acute schizophrenics, 8 and 12% among the biological relatives of the process schizophrenics, 13 to 20% among the biological relatives of the borderline schizophrenics, and approximately 2% among the biological relatives of the controls. An exact probability test reveals the difference in prevalence of doubtful borderline schizophrenia between the biological relatives of the acute schizophrenics and those of the controls is significant at the .04 level.

One should obviously not reach theoretically important conclusions on the basis of such a small sample and such marginal significance. I have submitted these data to fairly careful analysis because our initial inspection had suggested that the acute schizophrenias did not belong in our so-called "schizophrenic spectrum." Re-analysis suggests the deferment of decision—the acute schizophrenias may indeed be a part of the "schizophrenic spectrum."

A second group of studies which we conducted also suggests that borderline schizophrenia is a part of the schizophrenic spectrum. In this group of studies, called the "Adoptee Studies" (7, 8), we investigated the type and severity of psychopathology in a number of groups of subjects. For purposes of the present analysis, I shall confine myself to a discussion of two of these groups: the Index Group of individuals born to schizophrenics and adopted by parents who had never been psychiatrically diagnosed, and the Control Group of individuals born to biological parents who had never received a psychiatric hospitalization and who were reared by adopted parents who had likewise never received a psychiatric hospitalization.

These two groups of subjects, numbering 69 and 79 individuals, respectively, were interviewed by a psychiatrist who was blind as to the biological parents' diagnoses, and his clinical evaluations were blindly diagnosed. Analysis of the data revealed that there was an increased frequency of borderline or more severe schizophrenic psychopathology in the subjects in the Index Group, individuals whose biological parents were chronic or borderline schizophrenics. This finding not only suggests a genetic contribution to the etiology of the borderline schizophrenias but also suggests that borderline and chronic schizophrenia are related. As in the family study, we must—and have not yet—inspected the relationship of process and borderline-like schizophrenia in the biological parent to the diagnostic status of the child; we must see if process schizophrenic biological parents as well as borderline schizophrenic parents have borderline schizophrenic children.

Now, what about the schizoid disorders? Table I showed that the prevalence of schizoid states was the same among the biological relatives of the Index Adoptees and the Control Adopteees. Seemingly, therefore, the schizoid states are not related to process, acute and borderline schizophrenia. Re-analysis suggests that this may not be so. The reason is related to the method by which we selected our Controls. As mentioned, we found that some individuals chosen as Controls had schizophrenic-like psychopathology or were unavailable for interview and hence of uncertain diagnostic status. We eiminated such Controls on a post hoc basis, designating the remaining 24 as "screened" Controls; of these, 17 had diagnoses of mild or severe personality disorder. Only 7 were diagnosed as normal. Let us now compare the prevalence of schizoid psychopathology in the Index Group and compare it with the prevalence of such pathology in the three groups of controls. The findings are shown in Table III.

As may be seen, the significance of the differences between the Index and Control Groups increases with increased "purification" of the latter, reaching an exact probability of .08. The sample is very small, that is a

TABLE III

Prevalence of Schizoid Personality in the Biological and Adoptive Relatives of Schizophrenic Index and Control Proband

Group & Type of Relative	Number with Information Available	Number of Certain or doubtful Chronic or Borderline Schiz.	Number of Relatives not Certain or Doubtful Chronic or Borderline Schiz.	No. of Relatinves with Schizoid Personality
Biological Index	124	28	96	13 (13.5%)a
Biological Control	148	8	140	13 (9.2%)b
Screened Biological Controls	102	3	99	7 (7.1%)c
"Purified" Biological Controls	33	0	33	1 (3.0%)d

a Percent of these cases not clearly or doubtfully schizophrenic who are schizoid
b p<.2 Fisher exact probability test, all controls vs. index
c p<.1 Fisher exact probability test, screened controls vs. index
d p<.01 Fisher probability test, "purified" controls vs. index

post hoc analysis, and the probability fails to reach statistical significance, but the data looked at in this way *suggest* that, like the acute schizophrenias, the schizoid states may be part of the schizophrenic spectrum. This is of interest because other data suggest the same conclusion.

The adoptee studies shed further light on the relationship between the schizoid states and the rest of the schizophrenic spectrum. As part of the adoption studies, we investigated the psychiatric status of the biological co-parent (9) of the schizophrenic parents in the Index Group. We did this in order to determine if assortative mating, that is, matings between two schizophrenics had a differential effect on the outcome in the adopted-away offspring. If assortative mating did play a role, we would anticipate that individuals whose parents were both in the schizophrenic spectrum would have a greater risk of schizophrenic psychopathology than would individuals only one of whose parents were members of the spectrum. Having blindly diagnosed the psychiatric status of the co-parent, we investigated the relationship between his or her diagnosis and the psychiatric status of the offspring. If we examine those instances in which the co-parent was either schizoid or doubtfully schizophrenic and compare the offspring of these co-parents with those who are not in the schizophrenic spectrum, we obtain the data as shown in Table IV.

As may be seen, there is a significantly increased frequency of schizophrenic spectrum disorders among those instances in which assortative mating took place. Since this assortative mating included not only schizoids but doubtful schizophrenics as well, the conclusion cannot be

TABLE IV

Offspring Diagnosis as Spectrum or Not Spectrum According
to the Diagnosis of the Co-Parent When All Index
Parents are Chronic Schizophrenics

Co-parent diagnosis	Diagnosis of Offspring	
	Spectrum	Not spectrum
Spectrum	5 (6)*	3 (4)
Not spectrum	1	10 (11)

* Figures in parentheses include subjects whose diagnosis was called "doubtful" by one judge but "spectrum" or "not spectrum" by the other. One subject was called "doubtful" by both judges, and cannot be shown in the table.

Fisher Exact Probability Test:
  P=0.024 (Ss called "doubtful" by one judge excluded)
  P=0.015 (Ss called "doubtful" by one judge included)

drawn that schizoid states alone contribute to increased probability of schizophrenia in the offspring and are therefore members of the spectrum. These findings are compatible with the hypothesis that schizoid states are in the spectrum, but obviously do not constitute decisive data.

A third study (10) sheds additional light on the relationship of schizoid personality to the "true" schizophrenias. In this study, the Adoptive Parents' Study, we employed the variant of carefully evaluating the adopting parents of adult schizophrenics and comparing them with two other groups of parents. The first comparison group consisted of the biological parents of schizophrenics, individuals who had reared their own children. The second comparison group consisted of the biological parents of non-genetically produced retardates. The rationale was as follows: If schizophrenia were largely produced by psychopathology in the rearing parents, we would anticipate that the adopting parents of schizophrenics would demonstrate as much psychopathology as the biological parents of schizophrenics. Contrariwise, if schizophrenia were largely genetically transmitted, we would anticipate that the adopting parents of schizophrenics would show no more psychopathology than any individuals who had reared difficult children. It is for this reason that we employed a second comparison group, the biological parents of retardates. Since some psychopathology in rearing parents might be the reaction produced by rearing a difficult child, we wished to control for this effect as best we could by employing a group of parents who had

TABLE V

Consensus Diagnoses from Interview Data

| | PARENTS OF: | | |
	Adopted Schizophrenics	Biological Schizophrenics	Retardates
Chronic Schizophrenia	—	3	—
Acute Schizophrenia	1	—	—
Borderline Schizophrenia	—	—	—
Doubtful Schizophrenia	3	3	2
Schizoid Personality	—	9	3
Severe Personality Disorder (obsessive, hysterical, sociopathic)	1	5	1
Other Diagnoses + No Psychiatric Disorder	33	18	32

been forced to contend with considerable problems in rearing their children. All three groups of parents were administered structured psychiatric interviews and the data from these interviews, blinded so as not to reveal the group under investigation, was diagnosed by two independent raters. There were 19 subjects in each of the three groups, and hence 38 parents in each group. The results are shown in Table V. Now, if the diagnoses are collapsed into "schizoid" and "other" and the comparison groups are combined, the distribution is as shown in Table VI.

TABLE VI

| | PARENTS OF: | |
	Adopted Schizophrenics & Retardates	Biological Schizophrenics
Schizoid Personality	3	9
Other	73	29

$x^2 = 8.99$, df$=1$, P$<.01$

As may be seen, there is an increased frequency of schizoid personality only in the biological parents of the schizophrenics, and this increase is statistically significant. Interestingly enough, borderline and/or doubtful borderline schizophrenic diagnoses did not distinguish among the three groups. The fact that in this study schizoid states were increased and borderline states were not, while in the other studies borderline states were more discriminating, may only indicate that the boundaries between the two are unclear and that what is called borderline in one study may be called schizoid in another. This probable diagnostic blurring suggests the necessity of developing operational diagnostic criteria, an issue to which I will return.

To summarize the analyses so far, it has been argued the adoption studies demonstrate that the borderline schizophrenias are indeed members of the schizophrenic spectrum and suggest that the acute schizophrenias and schizoid disorders may be members of the spectrum as well. I would now like to turn to the question of a more formal definition and characterization of the borderline schizophrenic states.

The borderline states are currently undergoing a vogue, and non-causal reflection might lead one to believe that our findings suggest that all conditions designated as "borderline" bear a relationship to process schizophrenia. This is clearly not so. The descriptions of borderline states (and the word "state" may or may not imply schizophrenia) derive from a variety of sources.

These include groupings based on phenomenology, presumed and inferred psychodynamics, and ego structure. Before assuming that our findings have a bearing on these other groups, it is important to determine if our definition of borderline schizophrenia corresponds to others' definitions of "borderline states." As noted above, in our diagnostic evaluations of individuals as borderline schizophrenics, we started from the cluster of symptoms initially defined by Hoch and Polatin. However, few subjects met all their criteria, and we often had to make inferences concerning the probable presence of certain criteria. Since we employed global judgments and inferences, we cannot be sure that our diagnostic judgments were based exactly on those criteria which we had initially chosen. We may have in all probability employed different criteria with the passage of time. Since our diagnoses are reliable, that is, since we agreed, we are sure that we have defined an entity which is not process schizophrenia, which bears a resemblance to pseudo-neurotic schizophrenia, and which occurs with increased frequency among the relatives of chronic schizophrenics.

What we must now do is to abstract the criteria that we had employed and use these criteria to form an operational measure for the diagnosis of borderline schizophrenia. A start has been made in this direction. We have taken part of the borderline schizophrenia sample and abstracted the attributes we felt the members had in common. This technique is what in logic is called "ostensive definition." One specifies a number of exemplars of the type in question and then goes back to abstract the characteristics of the group so designated.

In order to determine if this abstracting has isolated the relevant criteria, we must now subject them to a test. In collaboration with Drs. Jean Endicott and Robert Spitzer, we are submitting other cases—not the ones we used for our ostensive definition—to raters who will note the number and pattern of the symptoms in the other case histories we have obtained. They will then employ decision rules we have provided which designate an individual as borderline schizophrenic or not depending on the number and distribution of his or her symptoms. If this operational method works, if the same individuals are picked by these raters on the basis of their decision rules as were picked by the clinicians on the basis of the global judgments, we will know that we have specified the cluster of signs and symptoms which we have tacitly employed. We then will have defined the signs and symptoms of a disorder which is neither process nor acute schizophrenia but which is markedly increased among the biological relatives of schizophrenics. It is important to realize that borderline schizophrenia as defined in these studies may not bear any relationship to what other clinicians have called borderline states or borderline schizophrenias. This brings us to an important nosological point.

We have already clinically identified a group of individuals whom we designate as "borderline schizophrenics" and whom we hope to be able to define in less impressionistic ways. But what if our group of individuals does not conclude with other groups designated "borderline" by others? Who was correct? It is obvious that anyone is entitled to list a group of signs and symptoms which he or she believes cluster together, and designate them as a syndrome. He is also entitled to call them by any name he chooses. It will be misleading, however, if he calls them by a name which implies a relationship to disorders to which they actually bear no relationship. He may, for example, notice that impulsivity, affective lability, and fluctuating reality testing seem to occur in the same individuals. If he calls people possessing these attributes "borderlines" and if the term "borderline" is regarded by many as a shorthand for "borderline schizophrenia," he is implying that these individuals either share a resemblance to or a causal relationship with true schizophrenia.

The adoption studies should in no way prevent other clinicians from studying such interesting symptom clusters. What they should do—for the moment—is form the basic criteria for defining borderline schizophrenia. If these criteria do not include affective lability, then affective lability may not be clustered with the other defining symptoms of borderline schizophrenia. The cluster of impulsivity, affective lability, and fluctuating reality testing might form a statistically recognizable group, but if it is not increased among the biological relatives of process or borderline schizophrenia, it is not appropriate to designate it as borderline schizophrenia and it is confusing to designate it as "borderline." To further demonstrate the meaningfulness of the syndrome, one would have to employ additional validating data. One might, for instance, find that individuals with the syndrome had similar histories or a similar response to treatment, or, as in the adoption studies, that similar clusters were found in genetically related individuals. But, to be repetitious, if these genetically related individuals are not schizophrenic, additional confusion will be engendered if these other clusters are labeled as borderlines or as borderline schizophrenics. If the adoption studies indicate that some symptomatic and behavioral clusters which have been designated as "borderline" in the past do not occur with increased frequency among the separately reared relatives of schizophrenics or only overlap borderline schizophrenia as defined by us, then the relationship of these clusters to borderline schizophrenia is at best partial.

I say "partial" because of an interesting theoretical possibility relating to the fact that some other psychiatric disorders appear to have genetic components and that the possibility of hybrid psychiatric illnesses exists. Studies utilizing the adoption technique have shown genetic contributions to criminality and sociopathy. What would happen, one wonders, if a schizophrenic were to mate with a sociopath? Would it be possible that the offspring might manifest characteristics of both disorders? In particular, might an individual manifest some borderline schizophrenic characteristics together with certain sociopathic ones such as affective lability and impulsivity? If this did occur on a reasonably reliable basis, one might then discover another syndrome which partially overlapped "borderline schizophrenia," as defined by us, whose symptoms clustered together consistently and which bore a genetic relationship to schizophrenia.

The existence of such a syndrome or, indeed, the possibility of such hybrids, remains to be documented. The possibility for its test does exist, however. The adoption study of the co-parents, mentioned earlier, showed the existence of assortative mating, and there was an increased tendency for the schizophrenic biological mothers of the adoptees to mate with sociopathic men. Inspection of these offspring may reveal that those individuals stemming from this hybrid parentage manifest characteristics of both diagnostic groups. This possibility remains to be examined. I have mentioned it to suggest that our findings in regard to borderline schizophrenia do not rule out the existence of other syndromes which differ in symptomatology but still have, for reasons such as I have mentioned, a relationship to true schizophrenia.

In summary, let me review what the adoption studies have accomplished in regard to the schizophrenia spectrum concept. They have documented a genetic contribution to the chronic and borderline schizophrenias; they have shown that the borderline schizophrenias are related to the chronic schizophrenias; and they have, in addition, provided some evidence that the acute schizophrenias and the schizoid states may also be related to the "true" schizophrenias. The data are stronger for the borderline schizophrenias and schizoid states; therefore, before the membership of the latter in the schizophrenic spectrum is seconded, additional confirmatory data are needed. Finally, these studies have not only documented the existence of a relationship between borderline schizophrenia(s) and chronic schizophrenias but have, by a logical bootstrap operation, helped us to define the characteristics of the borderline schizophrenias. This should be of considerable value in its own right, for only by breaking down this confusing group of disorders into relatively homogeneous groups can we hope to obtain meaningful data in regard to their natural history, pathogenesis, diagnosis, and response to treatment.

REFERENCES

1. Hoch, P., & Polatin, P. Pseudoneurotic forms of schizophrenia. *Psychiatric Quarterly,* 23, 248-276, 1949.
2. Kallman, F. J. *The Genetics of Schizophrenia.* Locust Valley, New York: J. J. Augustin, 1938.
3. Kretschmer, E. *Physique and Character.* New York: Harcourt, Brace & Co., 1923.
4. Kety, S. S., Rosenthal, D., Wender, P. H., & Schulsinger, F. The types and prevalence of mental illness in the biological and adoptive families of adopted schizophrenics. In Rosenthal, D., and Kety, S. S. (Eds.), *The Transmission of Schizophrenia.* Oxford: Pergamon Press, 1968, pp. 345-362.
5. Kety, S. S., Rosenthal, D., Wender, P. H., Schulsinger, F., & Jacobsen, B. Mental illness in the biological and adoptive families of adopted individuals who have become schizophrenic: A preliminary report based upon psychiatric interviews. In Fieve, R., Rosenthal, D., and Brill, H. (Eds.), *Genetic Research in Psychiatry.* Baltimore and London: The Johns Hopkins University Press, 1975, pp. 147-165.
6. McCabe, M. S., & Strömgren, E. Reactive psychoses. *Archives of General Psychiatry,* 32, 447-454, 1975.
7. Rosenthal, D., Wender, P. H., Kety, S. S., Schulsinger, F., Welner, J., & Ostergaard, L. Schizophrenics' offspring reared in adoptive homes. In *The Transmission of Schizophrenia,* op. cit., pp. 377-391.
8. Wender, P. H., Rosenthal, D., Kety, S. S., Schulsinger, F., & Welner, J. Crossfostering: A research strategy for clarifying the role of genetic and experiential factors in the etiology of schizophrenia. *Archives of General Psychiatry,* 30, 121-128, 1974.
9. Rosenthal, D. The concept of subschizophrenic disorders. In Fieve, R. R., Rosenthal, D., and Brill, H. (Eds.), *Genetic Research in Psychiatry.* Baltimore: The Johns Hopkins Press, 1975, pp. 199-208.
10. Wender, P. H. Schizophrenics' adopting parents: Psychiatric status. Paper read at the Annual Meeting of the American Psychiatric Association, Anaheim, California, May 1975.

7

Genetic Patterns as They Affect Psychiatric Diagnosis

GEORGE WINOKUR, M.D.

The most efficient way to make a diagnosis is by the use of pathogno-monic symptoms. These are few and far between in medicine and virtually non-existent in psychiatry. Pathognomonic signs do exist in medicine, e.g., the Kayser-Fleischer ring of hepatolenticular degeneration in Wilson's disease, the Bence-Jones protein in multiple myeloma, or an elevated T-4 in thyrotoxicosis. There are, however, few unequivocal pathophysiologic findings in psychiatric illness. As a consequence, we are confronted with making a diagnosis on the basis of the clinical picture, the course of the illness, response to various treatments, and the familial background. The vast bulk of the data in psychiatry is concerned with the clinical picture and the course of the illness. Treatment is a relatively new diagnostic tool; although there is an active attempt to make diagnoses on the basis of responses to various kinds of therapy, this methodology is still in its infancy.

As regards specific genetic or familial patterns in psychiatric illnesses, it has long been known that a number of such illnesses do cluster in families. In recent years, there has been an attempt to associate special familial patterns with other aspects of illnesses. A viable diagnosis at this point requires a highly significant clustering of specific types of clinical pictures with specific types of outcomes, responses to treatment, and familial patterns. If the correlations between all of these factors are highly significant, we could argue with reason that the syndrome in question is a specific illness. In this paper one of the tasks is to present the way or ways in which familial or genetic patterns may lead to more precision in practical clinical diagnoses.

GENETIC PATTERNS AS RELATED TO PRACTICAL DIAGNOSTIC PROBLEMS

On occasion, the clinical picture seen in a particular patient is so obscure that the patient does not fit into a clear and unequivocal diagnostic group. Obtaining a systematic family history may be of value in interpreting an ambiguous set of symptoms and in suggesting treatment. For example, the mixture of typical schizophrenic symptoms and affective symptoms often leads to confusion over appropriate diagnosis. Table 1 shows the results of two separate studies which bear on this point (14, 32). There are highly significant differences in family histories between chronic schizophrenic and affective disorder patients, with the former having many schizophrenic relatives and the latter having many affective disorder relatives (30).

TABLE 1

Familial Morbid Risks for Affective Disorder and Schizophrenia in Affective Disorder, Acute Schizophrenia and Chronic Schizophrenia

Probands	N	1° Relatives Affective Disorder		1° Relatives Schizophrenia	
Study 1					
Affective Disorder	325	13.50%		0.62%	
			P<.0005		P<.005
Chronic Schizophrenia	200	5.50%		2.11%	
Study 2					
Acute Schizophrenia	28	20.1%		5.5%	
			P<.025		P=N.S.*
Chronic Schizophrenia	25	4.5%		15.1%	

* $X^2 = 3.5803$, d.f. = 1, just misses significance at .05 level of confidence ($X^2 = 3.841$, d.f. = 1, p<.05).

Patients with clear and unmixed clinical pictures pose very few problems diagnostically. However, there are many patients who have acute schizophrenic illnesses. These patients frequently have many affective symptoms as well as delusions and hallucinations. Synonyms for acute schizophrenia are schizophreniform reaction, schizoaffective disorder, reactive psychosis, atypical psychosis, cycloid psychosis and psychogenic psychosis. The first two rows in Table 1 compare affective disorder and schizophrenic patients. There are notable differences in the family history between these two groups. The second two rows compare acute schizophrenics and chronic schizophrenics. The numbers here are smaller, but nevertheless a statistical difference does emerge. Acute schizophrenics have more affective disorder in their families than do chronic schizophrenics. Thus, in a patient with an admixture of affective and schizophrenic symptoms, the presence of a family history of affective disorder would lead one to consider the possibility that the acute schizophrenic, in fact, has a variant of affective disorder and, therefore, should be treated as a person with affective disorder rather than a person with schizophrenia. The treatments could be quite different. In addition, the discussion with the family about prognosis would be different.

It is interesting to note in Table 1 that the differences between affective disorder and chronic schizophrenia and between acute schizophrenia and chronic schizophrenia are both in the same direction. Familially, affective disorders and acute schizophrenia appear similar. Though these are separate studies, they are both blind as regards family history and they display some internal consistency.

Another study may be cited as showing the importance of the family history in predicting outcome. Winokur and Tsuang (34) published data on 62 recovered schizophrenics versus 61 non-recovered schizophrenics. The diagnoses were made 40 years ago by clinicians in a psychiatric hospital. In the group of recovered schizophrenics, there was a significantly increased likelihood of a clustering of remitting illnesses in the family.

It seems clear that the family history can be of some value in diagnosis. Of course, *it cannot be used instead of a good clinical evaluation,* but in the ambiguous case it may be of value in predicting outcome and planning treatment. Though these data are in favor of a relationship between schizoaffective disorder and affective disorder, the possibility remains that the former, in whole or in part, may be an autonomous third psychosis. Further family studies could settle this issue.

The Use of the Familial Psychiatric Background in Separating Out Homogeneous Illnesses in the Affective Disorders

There is a second consideration, perhaps more important than simply using family history for solving practical problems in diagnosis. It concerns whether genetic or familial patterns may be of value in separating out autonomous disease entities in psychiatry. It is conceivable that patients who are admitted for psychiatric care and presenting with essentially the same syndrome may be suffering from different disease processes. The syndrome is the final common pathway which brings the patient to the attention of the psychiatrist. However, the pathophysiology may not be homogeneous and the final common pathway may represent two or more specific illnesses. At present the closest we can come to the pathophysiology is the familial or genetic background. It is an etiology, but it is a distal etiology rather than a proximal one. The proximal etiology is the special pathophysiology itself. The distal etiology (genetic) indicates a biologic factor which evolves or develops into the syndrome. Nevertheless, a *different* set of familial findings in two groups of patients, both of whom manifest the same clinical picture, would be indicative of the fact that the illness is not a homogeneous entity.

That diagnostic homogeneity in psychiatric populations is absolutely necessary is self-evident. Without such homogeneity, it will not be possible to obtain specific proximal etiologies or effective treatments. The methodology for using the genetic or familial background to separate out homogeneous illnesses and ultimately to make a specific diagnosis is a complex one. Following is an outline of how this might be accomplished.

A Familial (Genetic) Methodology in Psychiatric Diagnosis

1. Accumulation of a group of patients with a homogeneous clinical picture and outcome.
2. Separation of these patients into subgroups on basis of specific variables, e.g., age of onset, sex, special clinical features.
3. Search for specific familial configurations of psychiatric illness in these subgroups.

or conversely

2a. Separate patients into subgroups on basis of different familial configurations of psychiatric illness.
3a. Search for special clinical or outcome variables in these subgroups.

4. Define subgroups in a reasonable fashion for further research.
5. Accomplish a family study in order to determine whether
   a. a specific kind of genetic transmission is present
   b. linkage exists between ill family members of the subgroup and known genetic markers
   c. association occurs between known genetic traits and the psychiatric illness which has been defined.

The last points 5, a, b, c are of importance as they provide validating evidence that the syndrome, in fact, is an autonomous disease.

The Division of the Affective Disorders into Bipolar and Unipolar Types

In a hospital that serves acute psychiatric patients, a large number of the admissions will be people who suffer from primary affective disorders. From one study of 1075 consecutive psychiatric admissions, 426 (40%) presented with affective syndrome, mania or depression (21). Clinically these patients were diagnosed as having neurotic depressions, psychotic depressions, manic-depressive illnesses and involutional depressions. Most of these patients had simple depressions, but 59 (14%) of the 426 were either manic at the time of admission or had been manic prior to admission. The depressive syndromes in the patients who had only depression are not easily differentiable on a clinical basis from the depressive syndromes seen in the patients who had a mania prior to admission. The important question is whether the members of this large group of affectively disordered patients are suffering from one or more diseases. As the clinical pictures of all these patients are rather similar, an appropriate way to answer this question would be to use a genetic or familial methodology.

In 1966, separate studies were presented concerning this matter by Angst in Zurich (1), Perris in Sweden (19) and Winokur and Clayton in St. Louis (30). Of interest is the fact that though a genetic methodology was used by all three of these groups, the specific methodologies differed.

Winokur and Clayton started with a group of 426 affectively disordered patients. They separated these patients into two subgroups. The first had a two-generation history of affective disorder, i.e., parent and proband or parent and child. They compared this subgroup with a family history negative subgroup which had no familial psychiatric illness of any type that could be gleaned from the history. All of the family histories were systematically obtained from the proband and usually from an accompanying relative. Table 2 gives some of the dif-

TABLE 2

Comparison of Family History Positive Probands (2 Generations
of Affective Disorder) with Family History
Negative Probands (No Family History of
Any Psychiatric Illness)

	FH—	FH+
N	129	112
Onset before 50	66%	75%
Proportion female	69%	65%
History of previous episode	57%	68%
Manic on admission	3%*	14%*

Depressive Symptoms in Non-Manic Patients

N	125	96
Retardation	46%	48%
Suicidal attempts in past or with present illness	17%	19%
Weight loss	60%	70%
Terminal insomnia	71%	76%
Self-deprecation	59%	61%

* Difference 3 vs. 14% p<.003.

ferences that were seen in comparing the group of patients that had no family history of psychiatric disorder with the group that had a family history of two generations of affective disorder. What is clear is the fact that those patients who had a two-generation history of affective disorder had a highly significant excess of admissions for mania. A comparison of the two groups as regards the frequencies of depressive symptoms showed no reliable differences. Thus, starting with a difference in familial transmission, we find that there is also a difference in the presence of a specific clinical finding. Mania is significantly more likely to be found in a family where there are two generations of affectively ill people than in a family where no other psychiatric illness exists. The depressive syndrome does not differ regardless of the kind of familial transmission. On the basis of differing familial transmissions, it was then

TABLE 3

A Comparison of Affective Illness in Family
Members of Manic Depressive (Bipolar)
vs. Depressive (Unipolar) Probands (3)

	PARENTS AND SIBS	
	Bipolar or manic	Depression only
Bipolar	3.7 % — 10.8 %	9.12% — 14.3 %
Depressive	0.29% — 0.35%	11.4 % — 14.2 %

TABLE 4

Familial Differences Between Manic-Depressive
Disease (Bipolar) and Depressive Disease

	Bipolar	Unipolar	P
Affective disorder in parent	52%	26%	.001
Two generation families	54%	32%	.01
Affective illness in parents or extended family	63%	36%	.0005
Mania in 1° relatives	3.7-10.8%	0.29-0.35%	

postulated that there were at least two kinds of affective disorder, manic-depressive disease and depressive disease.

Angst and Perris investigated the problem in a different way. They started with patients who had manias and depressions and compared these patients with those who had only depressions (3). Table 3 gives some of the data from these studies. It is clear that patients with manias *and* depressions have more relatives who have mania than do patients with *only* depressions. Perris termed those patients with manias and depressions as bipolar and those with only depressions as unipolar.

The result was essentially the same in all three studies. These and other data support the concept that there are two types of affective disorder, manic-depressive disease (bipolar) and depressive disease (unipolar) (4). Table 4 summarizes the familial differences between bipolar and unipolar affective disorders. Not only are more manics seen in the families of bipolar probands, but manic probands have a more extensive family history of affective illnesses than depressive probands.

Manic-Depressive Disease (Bipolar)

Winokur, Clayton and Reich (31) accomplished an intensive study of 61 manic patients. They found that in the families of manic patients there was a significant number of family members who had manias or mania and depression. There was also an equally large number of family members who had only depressions. Thus, a legitimate definition of manic-depressive disease (bipolar illness) is an illness seen in a patient who manifests manias and depression, or manias only, *or* who exhibits depressions only but comes from a family where mania exists. *The definition, in essence, becomes a familial one.*

In the group of manic patients studied by Winokur, Clayton and Reich (31), there was evidence that X-linkage was involved. In the families of these patients, significantly more women than men were affectively ill. The manic males had equal numbers of affectively ill brothers and sisters, but manic females had more affectively ill sisters. In this study, there was no instance of father to son transmission of affective illness. All of these points are in favor of a dominant X-linked transmission in manic-depressive disease.

Two large pedigrees were found where bipolar illness was assorting with color blindness, one protan, one deutan. In these two families, there was evidence that a presumptive manic-depressive locus was linked to the color blind locus. As the color blindness locus is on the X-chromosome, it provides further proof that manic-depressive illness is transmitted in a dominant X-linked fashion. Winokur and Tanna (33) also presented significant evidence favoring X-linkage in a set of families. There was a suggestion (not significant) in these data that there was specific linkage with the Xg^a blood locus, a blood group marker on the X-chromosome. Subsequent research by Mendlewicz, Fieve, Fleiss and Rainer (6, 16) enlarged on the linkage findings. These investigators studied a large number of pedigrees and showed linkage between the color blindness loci as well as linkage between the presumptive manic-depressive locus and the Xg^a locus. Table 5 presents the linkage material in tabular form. As part of their linkage study, Mendlewicz and Fleiss (16) also studied four informative kindreds of unipolar depression and protanopia as well as 12 pedigrees for unipolar depression and the Xg^a blood system. They found no

TABLE 5

Linkage Studies in Bipolar Affective Disorder

Study	Genetic Marker	Results
1. Winokur & Tanna (33)	Xgª	Report 3 pedigrees informative for linkage. In these, 10 children were compatible with X-linked transmission, one was incompatible. This difference is significant (2 of the 3 families suggest specific linkage with Xgª blood system. This was not significant, however).
2. Reich, Clayton & Winokur (21)	Red-green color blindness	Report 2 pedigrees, one with protan, the other with deutan color blindness. In each pedigree significant evidence of linkage with color blindness was found. Pedigrees suggest dominant inheritance.
3. Fieve, et al. (6)	Red-green color blindness	Report 8 pedigrees—4 with protan and 4 with deutan color blindness. Total of protan and deutan families gave significant evidence for linkage. Pedigrees fit a dominant inheritance.
4. Mendlewicz & Rainer (17)	Xgª	Report 23 kindreds for Xgª, linkage favored at odds of 900:1.
	Red-green color blindness	Report 17 informative kindreds for protan and deutan color blindness. Linkage between bipolar illness and deuteranopia favored at odds of 30,000:1. Linkage for protanopia, odds in favor, 5,000:1.

evidence for linkage between unipolar illness and either of these X-linked markers. The positive linkage findings for bipolar illness provided the impetus for a number of other studies to determine if, in fact, X-linkage was a means of transmission for manic-depressive illness. The studies by Goetzl et al. (9), Perris (20) and others presented reasonable findings indicating that father to son transmission did occur, in fact, in manic-depressive illness. These are summarized in Table 6. Thus, although the linkage studies are highly in favor of specific linkage with X-linked markers and, therefore, highly in favor of some bipolar patients having their illness transmitted in an X-linked fashion, it is necessary to state that X-linkage is not the only way in which manic-depressive illness is transmitted.

Fieve et al.'s study (6) is particularly important as this group of polar probands contains the probands who contributed to the positive finding of linkage between the manic-depressive disease locus and color

TABLE 6

Father-to-Son "Transmission" of Bipolar Affective Disorder:
Series Not Compatible with X-Linked Transmission as
the Sole Transmission Possibility

1. Perris (20)	In series of 138 bipolar probands, 13 11 father-son pairs.
2. Dunner, Gershon & Goodwin (5)	In 23 bipolar male patients, 4 had affectively ill fathers.
3. Goetzl, et al. (9)	In 39 bipolar families, 4 ill father-son pairs (no illness on maternal side).
4. Fieve, et al. (6)	In 120 bipolar probands, 13 ill father-son pairs (9 pairs no evidence of illness on maternal side).
5. Helzer & Winokur (10)	Of 30 male manics, 8 affectively ill mothers (41%), and 1 affectively ill father (5%); in another ill father-ill son pair, considerable affective disorder existed on the maternal side of the family.
6. Von Greiff, McHugh & Stokes (25)	In 16 male probands, 4 ill father-son pairs with no illness on maternal side; 3 ill father-son pairs did have illness on maternal side.

blindness loci, as well as the probands who show father to son transmission. An appropriate evaluation of the material would indicate that there are at least two kinds of transmission in manic-depressive illness, one of which is X-linkage.

Further Data Related to X-linkage

The question of whether X-linkage occurs in bipolar illness is a matter of extreme importance. A positive finding proves the presence of a genetic factor in manic-depressive disease beyond a shadow of a doubt. It proves the opportunity to determine a high-risk group and to engage in biologic studies of this group. Thus, with the presence of X-linkage certain kinds of families could be found which show the hallmarks of this kind of transmission. Such hallmarks would be the absence of father to son transmission in the pedigree and the transmission of illness to sons from the mother or at least the maternal side of the family. Such families would contain more affectively ill women than affectively ill males. In some families where color blindness was also assorting, one could specifically determined which person was likely to become ill. Likewise, if the data were positive for linkage of bipolar illness with the Xg^a blood system, families could be found where specific people would be considered at high risk for affective illness. It would then be possible to study the biology of these people long before they became ill because one could predict illness in a specific person. Finally, the demonstration of X-linkage in some cases, but not in others, would indicate genetic heterogeneity in bipolar illness. Such heterogeneity might manifest itself in a different progression of symptoms or in different responses to specific treatments or in different biologic findings.

To determine linkage of bipolar illness with a known genetic locus on the X-chromosome requires a very specific way of approaching the problem. In families where father to son transmission occurs, it would be inappropriate to look for such a transmission. Only in families where the transmission appears to be X-linked, i.e., is consistent with the expectations of X-linkage, could one make the next step. This next step obviously would be to search for linkage with specific markers, i.e., such markers as color blindness or the Xg^a blood system. In fact, this has been done and the data support X-linkage very significantly. There are some circumstances which support the validity of linkage studies in manic-depressive illness: Firstly by their very nature the linkage studies are done blindly; secondly, the findings are positive even though the original groups of probands probably contain more than one type of transmission; thirdly, the findings of linkage are positive in the face of the possibilities that some of the familial affective states may be related to alcoholism rather than manic-depressive illness. It is clear that depressives are frequently seen in the families of alcoholics. This would produce considerable noise in the system but the linkage data are still positive. Finally, the findings are positive even though some relatives may appear to be negative for affective illness because they have not passed the age of risk. However, as has been noted above, there are also good data in the literature, i.e., the presence of ill father to ill son pairs, which support a non-X-linked type of transmission.

As the linkage findings support the concept of genetic heterogeneity in bipolar illness, X-linkage must be taken into account before one can consider other types of transmission in groups of probands. There has been some interest in the possibility of a polygenic transmission in bipolar illness but it is questionable whether this could be proven until the groups are divided according to the X-linked type and the non-X-linked type. It is entirely possible that polygenicity is involved even in the X-linked type of illness. All that has been demonstrated by the linkage studies is that an X-linked factor is present in some families. For further

TABLE 7

Sex Ratios in Bipolar Series

	N	Proportion Female
Angst, et al. (2)	393	71%
Perris (19)	138	59%
Winokur (26)	89	61%
Iowa 500 (28)	109	58%
Stenstedt (23)	63	54%
Mendlewicz & Rainer (17)	134	58%
Lundquist (13)	103	54%
Woodruff, et al. (35)	19	53%
James & Chapman (11)	46	54%

genetic or biologic studies, such families must be separated from the non-X-linked type of families. This would be a necessity before studies concerning the possibility of polygenic transmission were embarked upon.

It may be possible to evaluate the amount of X-linkage in the universe of bipolar patients. Clearly some estimate is necessary regarding how many families might be expected to show X-linkage and how many would be not expected to show this. Some of the epidemiologic data that are available in the literature may shed some light on this question.

Numerous series of manic or bipolar probands have been reported in the literature, and many of them show an excess of female over male patients. This finding would be expected if X-linkage were involved in all or even some of the families of the probands. Table 7 shows the proportion of females in various studies which have been reported in the literature. It is noteworthy that all these studies show the proportion of females larger than that of males. The female proportions vary between 53 and 71%. Assuming both a low gene frequency for a presumptive bipolar gene *and* dominant X linkage as the sole means of transmission, one would expect that almost 67% of the patients who showed the illness should be female. As the gene frequency becomes higher, there is an attrition of the 67% finding so that if the gene frequency of a dominant X-linked gene were 100%, there should be a 50-50 proportion of males and females (15, Fig. 11). This is the same sex ratio, $M:F = 1:1$, that would be expected in autosomal transmission. Certainly the sex ratios in the bipolar series do not conform to either an autosomal transmission or an X-linked dominant transmission with a

TABLE 8

M:F Ratio in Population
First Admission Bipolar Illness

	M	F	%F
Spicer, et al. (22) England & Wales 1965 & 1966	1056	1500	59%
Denmark 1967; 1968; 69/70; 71/72	159	207	57%

Lifetime Morbid Risk

James & Chapman (11) New Zealand	—	—	57%

low gene frequency. The data from reported series in Table 7 may be highly biased as they may reflect simply who gets treated in hospitals. One would like to have a figure that was relevant to the population. In other words, what would the female-male ratio be for bipolar illness in the general population?

One may approach this by looking at national figures and these are available for Denmark, England and Wales, and New Zealand (11, 18, 22). Table 8 presents sex ratio material on first admissions and lifetime morbid risks of bipolar illness. It is clear from these data that the proportion that are female vary in these large samples between 57 and 59%. This does not fulfill the 67% criterion which would be necessary to consider that all bipolar illness is transmitted in an X-linked dominant fashion. To achieve a proportion of females of 59%, assuming only an X-linked type of transmission were involved, would mean that the gene frequency for bipolar illness would have to be around .60 (15). This would mean that 60% of the males in the population should be ill. In fact, in a study from Bornholm Island, Denmark (8), the male population frequency for manic-depressive illness is closer to 1% than to 60%.

Taking into account the linkage studies which suggest X-linkage and heterogeneity, it is necessary then to postulate two types of transmission in the population to account for the 57% to 59% proportion of ill females. If in fact these figures do reflect the true sex differential in bipolar illness, one may use the material from the British First Admissions for Mania (22) and calculate the percentage of the entire group which are X-linked.

BRITISH FIRST ADMISSIONS FOR MANIA
1965-1966

Males 1056; Females 1500; Total 2556
(a = Number of patients who are X-linked)

$$.67a + .5 \ (2556 - a) = 1500$$
$$a = \frac{222}{.17} = 1306$$

non a = 2556 — 1306 = 1250
of the entire group of 2556, 1306 are
X-linked

$$\frac{1306}{2556} = 51\%$$

The above calculation shows that 51% of our bipolar patients are probably subject to X-linked transmission. It is based on the idea that in one kind of transmission, dominant X-linkage, 67% of the bipolars will be female; in the other kind of transmission, autosomal, 50% of the bipolars will be female. A necessary question is whether or not the first admissions in Great Britain and Denmark actually reflect the sex differential in the population. In one study it was noted that females were likely to be admitted earlier than males (31). This could reflect the possibility that women are more likely to seek help. However, a subsequent and unpublished larger study on the difference in the period between onset of illness and hospitalization in males versus females indicated that there is no evidence that females are likely to be admitted earlier than males (see Table 9).

TABLE 9

Length of Illness Prior to Index
Admission (94 Manics)

	Male	Female
N	36	58
1 Month or Less	69%	62%
3 Months	11%	12%
6 Months	11%	10%
1 Year or More	6%	15%

$X^2 = 2.096$, df$=3$,
p$=$N.S.

There is one study of a total population which offers some data on the male/female breakdown of bipolars and manics. This is concerned with a cohort of patients from Iceland. In a personal communication from Dr. T. Helgason who carried out this epidemiological and follow-up investigation of the cohort, 37 patients were identified as having mania or manias and depressions; of these 22 (59%) were female and 15 (41%) were male. Dr. Helgason has kindly given us permission to quote these data.

A possible explanation which has been offered to explain the increased proportion of females in bipolar illness is that for some biological reason females with the same gene or genes are more likely to become ill. There are no data which answer this question directly. What would be necessary would be a group of bipolar patients who were members of same sex dizygotic pairs. If both the male and female pairs had equal concordance, one would not be able to say that women were more likely to become ill with bipolar illness than men. Kringlen (12, Table 29) summarizes some material on this point. Unfortunately, it is difficult to determine whether or not these are bipolar patients alone or unipolar and bipolar patients mixed. Nevertheless, from the material one can see that the percentage of female dizygotic pairs who were concordant is 22-29%; the percentage of concordance for male dizygotic pairs is 17-33%. There is no obvious difference in propensity for concordance between these two groups.

One, then, is left with the conclusion that, considering the linkage data, it is highly likely that there is genetic heterogeneity. Using epidemiological material, it is possible to calculate that slightly over half of the bipolar patients in the population will have their illness transmitted in an X-linked fashion.

The Division of Unipolar Depression into Depression
Spectrum Disease and Pure Depressive Disease

The major portion of affectively disordered patients who are seen in a hospital are unipolar. The question then arises as to whether unipolar depression is a homogeneous illness or whether it is comprised of two or more autonomous entities.

The first indication that the latter might be the case came as a result of a study of 100 rigorously diagnosed depressive probands (29). In this group of 100, all bipolar patients were excluded, as were any depressive

TABLE 10

Depression Risks for Parents and Sibs of Early ($<$ 40)
and Late ($>$ 40) Onset Depressive Patients

	Number at Risk	Number Depressed	Morbid Risk
Early Onset			
Mothers	51	12	24%
Fathers	49	4	8%
Sisters	28	8	29%
Brothers	24	3	13%
Total	152	27	18%
Late Onset			
Mothers	45	6	13%
Fathers	40	5	13%
Sisters	60	9	15%
Brothers	65	9	14%
Total	210	29	14%

patients who had a family history of bipolar illness. After considerable
evaluation of the data, it became clear that early onset depressives had a
markedly different family history than late onset depressives. Table 10
gives this material. The female relatives in the early onset group are
more likely ill with depression than the females of the late onset group,
but this misses significance. In the early onset group, it is clear that
mothers and sisters have a significantly higher morbid risk for depression
($p < .025$) than do fathers and sons. In the late onset group, both male
and female relatives have an almost equal morbid risk.

Table 11 shows the risks for alcoholism or antisocial personality in the
early onset versus the late onset depressive groups. From Table 11, it
can be seen that 15% of the parents and sibs at risk of the early onset
group have alcoholism and/or antisocial personality, whereas only 2%
of the late onset group show this finding in their relatives. This is a
highly significant difference ($\chi^2 = 15.36$, $df = 1$, $p < .005$ with Yates cor-
rection).

One may also compare total illness in the two groups. Total illness
refers to alcoholism, antisocial personality and depression. The difference
between the two groups is highly significant ($p < .0005$). There is a

TABLE 11

Alcoholism and/or Antisocial Personality in Parents
and Sibs of Early Onset ($<$ 40) vs. Late Onset
($>$ 40) Depressive Patients

	Number of Parents and Sibs at Risk	Number with Alcoholism and/or Antisocial Personality	Proportion Ill
Early Onset (N=54)	152	23	15%
Late Onset (N=46)	210	5	2%

TABLE 12

Paternal Alcoholism in Depressive Patients
(5 Studies Pooler, 1165 Probands)

	Alcoholic Fathers of Male Probands	Alcoholic Fathers of Female Probands
Age Onset, Proband		
$<$20 — 39 (E.O.)	10%	14%
40 — 60+ (L.O.)	4%	5%

trend for the early onset group to have depressed parents and sibs accompanied with the late onset group, but this is not significant. Obviously, then, the significant difference between the two groups is associated with alcoholism and the antisocial personality which is seen in male relatives of early onset depressives.

Six studies have been reported which deal with the same kind of data (27). The results are: a) 6 out of the 6 studies show that familial affective disorder is more frequent in early onset than late onset probands; b) 6 out of the 6 studies showed that alcoholism in relatives is more frequent in early onset than late onset probands; c) in 5 out of the 6 studies male relatives of late onset male probands had amounts of affective disorder equal to or greater than female relatives; d) in 5 out of the 6 studies female relatives are more likely depressed than male relatives in families of early onset female probands.

These six studies comprise 1255 probands. They sample patients who were admitted to hospital at diverse periods of time. One of the studies deals with outpatients, one deals with patients admitted to a separate medical facility from the other five.

Table 12 shows pooled data encompassing 1165 probands and is concerned with the presence of paternal alcoholism in groups separated by sex and age of onset (27). It is clear that there is a highly significant difference in the early onset group versus the late onset group. Early onset males are more likely to have alcoholic fathers than late onset males ($p < 0.05$). For females the significance is much higher with the early onset female probands having more alcoholic fathers than the late onset female probands ($p < 0.0005$).

In light of these findings two kinds of illnesses were postulated. First of these was depression spectrum disease, the prototype of which was the early onset female. Such a patient was very likely to have alcoholism and/or antisocial personality in her family. Her female relatives were more likely depressed than her male relatives. The total illness (alcoholism, antisocial personality, depression) was around 23% in first-degree relatives. The other prototype was considered the late onset male who manifested what we termed pure depressive disease. In the case of late onset male, alcoholism was a negligible factor in the family, males and females were likely to be equally ill with depression, and the total amount of illness was around 13%.

One question which was important was whether or not there was any correlation between the age of onset in the depressed patient and the depressed relatives. Table 13 indicates that the early onset probands were likely to have as many late onset depressive relatives as early onset relatives (p < 0.025).

TABLE 13

Relationship of Age of Onset in Depressive
Probands vs. Depressive Parents and Sibs

| | PARENTS AND SIBS | | |
	Early Onset	Late Onset	Total
Early Onset	15 (8)	12 (8)	27
Probands			
Late Onset	6 (1)	23 (10)	29

Early Onset <40; Late Onset >40.
Numbers in parenthesis refer to parents only.

Of interest is the fact that further confirmation of the above findings comes from an independent study in Greece. Frangos, et al. (7) have shown that early onset unipolar depressives are significantly more likely to have relatives with psychopathic personalities than are late onset unipolar depressives. Also, in the families of the early onset patients, females are more frequently likely to suffer from depression than the female relatives of late onset cases.

The Appropriate Definition of Depression
Spectrum Disease and Pure Depressive Disease

It is clear that depression spectrum disease is more likely seen in a female than a male, and more likely seen in early onset patients. To use a definition of depression spectrum disease which encompasses these points is unwieldy. Further, from Table 13 one may note that the depressed relatives of the early onset patients are equally likely to have a late onset as an early onset (before and after 40). There is a logical problem in using the age of onset as a defining factor. An early onset female could well be used as a depression spectrum disease proband; however, if her relative had an illness after 40, one would question the validity of this break. In fact, this late onset relative could be used as a pure depressive disease proband. For these reasons, we have been concerned with a reasonable and workable definition of depression spectrum disease. As a significant qualitative and quantitative difference seems to be the presence or absence of alcoholism in a family, *we have defined depression spectrum disease as an illness in any patient who had a rigorously diagnosed depression and has an alcoholic or antisocial member in the first-degree relative group.* Certainly, from the family studies, the presence of alcoholism or antisocial personality in a first-degree relative would be associated with being an early onset female depressive but this would not be an invariable finding. There would be too much overlap with other types of patients. Thus, the definition of depression spectrum disease is dependent on the familial disease pattern as well as the clinical picture in the proband.

A Linkage Study of Depression Spectrum Disease

Having evolved a workable definition of depression spectrum disease, it then became possible to push the investigation further by use of a linkage methodology. Appropriate groupings were made in the following manner. A proband could be admitted for either alcoholism or depression and if a first-degree family member of such a proband had one of the other illnesses, i.e., antisocial personality, alcoholism or depression, this kind of finding defined a family with depression spectrum disease. All first-degree family members were then interviewed and blood was drawn in order to make specific determination of various genetic markers. Another type of family was also collected. A family in which a proband had depression and a first-degree family member also had depression was used to define pure depressive disease. Such a pure depressive disease family by definition could not have had alcoholism or antisocial personality in a first-degree family member.

By the nature of the linkage study, blindness is accomplished automatically. Thus, a family is interviewed and diagnoses are made prior to the time that any knowledge has been obtained on the marker systems. The people determining the markers know nothing about the diagnosis, and the people making the diagnoses know nothing about the markers.

For depression spectrum disease, a total of 68 Caucasian individuals (39 males, 29 females) were collected (24). Fourteen different subships were represented by these 68 individuals. The subjects were interviewed and diagnoses were made according to rigorous criteria. Blood was drawn and sent to a marker laboratory. Diagnoses were as follows in the subships: alcoholism, 21; antisocial personality, 2; depression, 16; for a total of 39. All of these people were considered to have the same illness which, however, manifested itself differently in separate individuals. This manifestation was to a large extent dependent on sex, with the female sibs usually showing depression and the male sibs showing alcoholism and antisocial personality. Five subjects had other diagnoses, two with anxiety neurosis, one with hysteria, and two with undiagnosed psychiatric illness. Twenty-four subjects were considered normal.

The following genetic markers were determined for each individual: 1) ABO, 2) Rh, 3) Kell, 4) MNSs, 5) P, 6) Duffy, 7) Xg, 8) Kidd, 9) Lutheran, 10) Red cell acid phosphatase, 11) Adenosine deaminase, 12) Adenylate Kinase, 13) Glutamic pyruvic transaminase, 14) Phosphoglucomutase, 15) 6-phospho-gluconate dehydrogenase, 16) Group specific protein, 17) α-haptoglobin, 18) Third component of complement, 19) Hemoglobin β, 20) Transferrin.

Linkage was determined in an initial workup by the use of the sib pair method of Penrose. With this method each sib in the study is scored as being alike or unlike for the genetic marker and for illness (in this case, depression spectrum disease). Entries were made into a 2 x 2 table. Each box has a specific kind of an entry. Sib pairs are evaluated as to whether they were like for illness, like for marker, *or* unlike for illness, unlike for marker, *or* like for illness, unlike for marker, *or* unlike for illness, like for marker. If there is an excess number of pairs in the like-like and the unlike-unlike groups as compared to the two remaining groups, it would be considered evidence in favor of linkage. Using this method which is the least powerful statistically of all of the linkage methods, we found evidence in favor of linkage of depression spectrum disease with the third component of complement (C3) and the α-haptoglobin loci (α-Hp). When normals and other psychiatric illness are considered as a normal group and compared with a depression spectrum group (depression or alcoholism or antisocial personality), the level of significance for linkage with C3 is $p < .005$ and the level of significance for linkage with haptoglobin is $p < .005$. The sib pair data are presented in Table 14.

It is always possible that an association of the marker with the disease could give the impression of linkage where none exists. "Association" occurs when two presumably separate genetic traits have a non-random occurrence together in a population. It is most likely explained by pleiotropic effects of a single gene. In fact, there is no evidence that patients with depression spectrum disease are more or less likely to have any of the specific phenotypes of these two marker systems, C3 and α-haptoglobin.

The finding of *two* significantly positive relationships that indicate linkage of depression spectrum disease with genetic markers indicates a problem. If *one* had been found, we could say with some reason that linkage had occurred. Finding *two* makes the situation more problematic. It is possible that there is linkage with two markers. It is also possible that one of them, though of high significance, is really only a chance finding. There is a methodology for determining the meaning of the two positive findings. Material is available from parents as well as sibs. By the use of the lod score method and a more precise statistical evaluation of linkage, and with the addition of new data (from the extended families), it is quite possible that one of the positive findings will drop out and the other will become even more positive.

Suffice it to say that at this time the material is suggestive of linkage with one or both of the systems, C3 and α-haptoglobin.

If the linkage study continues to fulfill its promise, we will be able to

TABLE 14

Sibpair Analysis for α-Haptoglobin and Third
Component of Complement with Relationship
to Depression Spectrum Disease

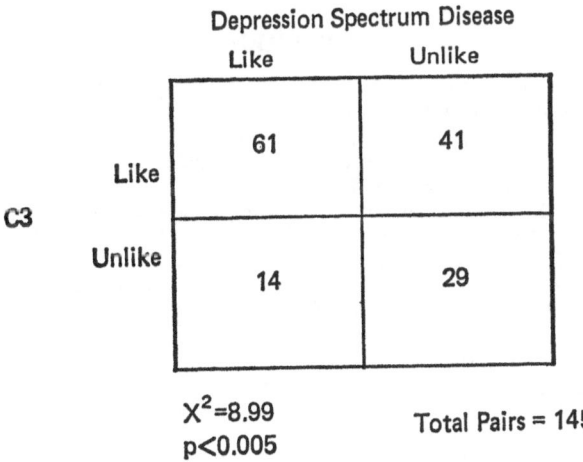

Depression Spectrum Disease

		Like	Unlike
	Like	57	36
α Haptoglobin	Unlike	22	40

$X^2 = 9.91$
$p < 0.005$ Total Pairs = 155

Depression Spectrum Disease

		Like	Unlike
	Like	61	41
C3	Unlike	14	29

$X^2 = 8.99$
$p < 0.005$ Total Pairs = 145

make a number of statements. The data from such a linkage study would be in favor of: 1) heterogeneity of unipolar depression, and 2) the presence of a specific and genetic illness which manifests itself usually as depression in women and alcoholism or antisocial personality in men.

CONCLUSIONS

The point of this odyssey through the affective disorders is to indicate that genetic principles have a significant role in elucidating diagnostic problems. Through the use of genetic variables, it has been possible to separate bipolar from unipolar affective disorder. With this accomplished, it has certainly been reasonable to investigate these two groups using other methods, namely neurochemical and electrophysiological. The finding of groups of affective disorders, which are considerably more homogeneous than have been considered in the past, has made it possible to search for and find specific biological correlates of these two illnesses.

Using a similar methodology, it has been possible to delineate two types of unipolar disorders—depression spectrum disease and pure depressive disease. An initial workup using a linkage methodology has suggested that these two unipolar illnesses are in fact distinct entities. Should the findings be expanded and replicated, we will be able to say that three types of affective disorders have been discovered, where in the past only one was presumed to have existed.

REFERENCES

1. Angst, J. Zur Atiologie und Nosologie endogener Depressiver Psychosen. *Monogr. Neurol. Psychiat.*, 113, 1, 1966.
2. Angst, J., Baastrup, P., Grof, P., Hippius, H., Poldinger, W., & Weis, P. The course of monopolar depression and bipolar psychoses. *Psychiatr. Neurol. Neurochir.*, 76, 489-500, 1973.
3. Angst, J., & Perris, C. Nosology of endogenous depression, a comparison of the findings of two studies. *Arch. Psychiat. Nervekr.*, 210, 373-386, 1968.
4. Dorzab, J., Baker, M., Cadoret, R., & Winokur, G. Depressive Disease: Familial psychiatric illness. *American Journal of Psychiatry*, 127, 1128-1133, 1971.
5. Dunner, D., Gershon, E., & Goodwin, F. Heritable factors in the severity of affective illness. Presented at 123rd Ann. Meet., APA, San Francisco, 1969.
6. Fieve, R., Mendlewicz, J., Rainer, J., & Fleiss, J. A dominant X-linked factor in manic-depressive illness: studies with color blindness. In Fieve, R., Rosenthal, D., & Brill, H. (Eds.), *Genetic Research in Psychiatry*. Baltimore: Johns Hopkins University Press, 1975.
7. Frangos, E., Christodoulidis, H., Tsitouridis, E., & Papadopoulos, K. Observations upon patients suffering from unipolar and bipolar affective disorders, presented at Hellenic Congress in Neurology & Psychiatry, Athens, Greece, October 29-November 3, 1975.

8. Fremming, K. *The Expectation of Mental Infirmity in a Sample of the Danish Population*. Occasional papers on eugenics, No. 7. London: Cassell & Co., Ltd., 1951.
9. Goetzl, U., Green, R., Wybow, P., & Jackson, R. X-linkage revisited. *Archives of General Psychiatry*, 31, 665-672, 1974.
10. Helzer, J., & Winokur, G. A family interview study of male manic depressives. *Archives of General Psychiatry*, 31, 73-77, 1974.
11. James, N., & Chapman, C. A genetic study of bipolar affective disorder. *British Journal of Psychiatry*, 126, 449-456, 1975.
12. Kringlen, E. *Heredity and Environment in the Functional Psychoses*. London: Wm. Heinemann Medical Books, 1967.
13. Lundquist, G. Prognosis and course in manic-depressive psychoses. *Acta Psychiatrica Neurologica Scandinavica* (Suppl. 13), 1945.
14. McCabe, M., Fowler, R., Cadoret, R., & Winokur, G. Familial differences in schizophrenia with good and poor prognosis. *Psychological Medicine*, 1, 326-332, 1971.
15. McKusick, V. *On the X Chromosome of Man*. Washington, D.C.: American Institute of Biological Sciences, 1964.
16. Mendlewicz, J., & Fleiss, J. Linkage studies with X chromosome markers in bipolar (manic depressive) and unipolar (depressive) illness. *Biological Psychiatry*, 9, 261-294, 1974.
17. Mendlewicz, J., and Rainer, J. Morbidity risk and genetic transmission in manic depressive illness. *American Journal of Human Genetics*, 26, 692-701, 1974.
18. National Health Service of Denmark, Medical Report II, fiscal year 1967/68, 1970/71, 1972/73, Copenhagen (1973, 1974, 1975).
19. Perris, C. (Ed.). A study of bipolar (manic-depressive) and unipolar recurrent depressive psychoses. *Acta Psychiatrica Scandinavica*, 42 (Suppl. 194), 1966.
20. Perris, C. Abnormality on paternal and maternal sides: Observations in bipolar (manic depressive) and unipolar depressive psychoses. *British Journal of Psychiatry*, 118, 207-210, 1971.
21. Reich, T., Clayton, P., & Winokur, G. Family history studies V. The genetics of mania. *American Journal of Psychiatry*, 125, 1358-1369, 1969.
22. Spicer, C., Hare, E., & Slater, E. Neurotic and psychotic forms of depressive illness: Evidence from age-incidence in a national sample. *British Journal of Psychiatry*, 123, 535-541, 1973.
23. Stenstedt, Å. A study in manic depressive psychosis. *Acta Psychiatrica Neurologica Scandinavica* (Suppl. 79), 1952.
24. Tanna, V., Winokur, G., Elston, R., & Go, R. A linkage study of depression spectrum disease: The use of the sib-pair method. *Neuropsychobiology*, 2:52-62, 1976.
25. Von Grieff, H., McHugh, P., & Stokes, P. The familial history in 16 males with bipolar manic-depressive illness. In Ficve, A., Rosenthal, D., and Brill, H. (Eds.), *Genetic Research in Psychiatry*. Baltimore: Johns Hopkins University Press, 1975.
26. Winokur, G. Genetic findings and methodological considerations in manic depressive disease. *British Journal of Psychiatry*, 117, 267-274, 1970.
27. Winokur, G. The division of depressive illness into depression spectrum disease and pure depressive disease. *International Pharmacopsychiatry*, 9, 5-13, 1974.
28. Winokur, G. The Iowa 500: Heterogeneity and course in manic-depressive illness (bipolar). *Comprehensive Psychiatry*, 16, 125-131, 1975.
29. Winokur, G., Cadoret, R., Baker, M., & Dorzab, J. Depression spectrum disease versus pure depressive disease: Some further data. *British Journal of Psychiatry*, 127, 75-77, 1975.

30. Winokur, G., & Clayton, P. Family history studies. I. Two types of affective disorders separated according to genetic and clinical factors. In Wortis, J. (Ed.), *Recent Advances in Biological Psychiatry*, Vol. 9. New York: Plenum Publishing Corp., 1967. (Presented at the 21st Annual Convention and Scientific Program of the Society of Biological Psychiatry, Washington, D.C., June, 1966).

31. Winokur, G., Clayton, P., & Reich, T. *Manic Depressive Illness*. St. Louis: C. V. Mosby Co., 1969.

32. Winokur, G., Morrison, J., Clancy, J., and Crowe R. The Iowa 500. II. A blind family history comparison of mania, depression and schizophrenia. *Archives of General Psychiatry*, 27, 462-464, 1972.

33. Winokur, G., & Tanna, V. Possible role of X-linked dominant factor in manic-depressive disease. *Diseases of the Nervous System*, 30, 89, 1969.

34. Winokur, G., & Tsuang, M. A clinical and family history comparison of good outcome and poor outcome schizophrenia. *Neuropsychobiology*, 1, 59-64, 1975.

35. Woodruff, R., Guze, S., & Clayton, P. Unipolar and bipolar primary affective disorder. *Brit. J. Psychiat.*, 119, 33-38, 1971.

8

The Vulnerable Brain: Biological Factors in the Diagnosis and Treatment of Depression

H. M. van Praag, M.D.

The following abbreviations are used in this paper:

α-MT	*α-methyl-p-tyrosine*	5-HTP	*5-hydroxytryptophane*
CA	*catecholamines*	HVA	*homovanillic acid*
CNS	*central nervous system*	MA	*monoamines*
CSF	*cerebrospinal fluid*	MAO	*monoamine oxidase*
DA	*dopamine*	MHPG	*3-methoxy-4-hydroxyphenyl-*
DOPAC	*3,4-dihydroxyphenylacetic acid*		*glycol*
DOPS	*dihydroxyphenylserine*	NA	*noradrenaline*
5-HIAA	*5-hydroxyindoleacetic acid*	pcpa	*p-chlorophenylalanine*
5-HT	*5-hydroxytryptamine (serotonin)*	VMA	*vanillylmandelic acid*

1. Imperfections of Psychiatric Diagnosis

Classification: Foundation of Diagnosis

Psychiatrists can lay no claim to a rich tradition in classification. They have long looked down on classification as a futile activity and a dangerous one to boot, one suggesting that a "labeling" of patients disregards that which is "essential" for them. This view is, of course, untenable. A scientific study should be preceded by a classification of the phenomena on which it focuses. Classification is the foundation of diagnosis and, without adequate diagnosis, treatment as well as research inevitably gives botched results.

153

Few psychiatrists are still openly opposed to this view today. The classification system available to them, however, is not a sound one. As compared with other medical disciplines, psychiatry has obviously lagged behind in this respect. I shall discuss a number of factors which make psychiatric classification imperfect and obscure.

Two-Dimensional Diagnosis

Psychiatric classification might be based on three pillars: symptomatology, aetiology and course. In actual practice, however, systematic use of each of these three is rare. For example, the term "endogenous depression" implies certain indications of the aetiology of this depression and of its symptomatology, but gives no information on its course. Another example: the term "unipolar depression" is indicative of a certain symptomatology with a certain course, but gives no information on the aetiology of this depression.

Two-dimensional diagnosis would be justifiable only if the description of two criteria would virtually establish the character of the third criterion. This is not true. Take the example of a unipolar depression. This involves a vital depressive syndrome with a phasic course, without (hypo)manic periods. But this description by no means establishes its aetiology. The latter may involve not only a pronounced hereditary factor, but equally a certain personality structure and/or a given situation of life. The latter may again and again create the conditions required for a depressive episode.

Another example: a diagnosis such as psychogenic schizophrenia gives no information on the course of the condition. Yet, given a particular aetiology and a particular syndrome, the course is not predetermined. Several different courses are possible: an acute course with complete recovery to the premorbid level, a recurrent course with complete recovery after each phase, and a recurrent course with gradual deterioration of the personality.

Finally a concept such as pre-oedipal neurosis with recurrent decompensations is an example of a dynamic diagnosis in which aetiology and course are indicated but symptomatology ignored.

One-Dimensional Diagnosis

If two-dimensional diagnosis is inadequate, the one-dimensional diagnosis is even more unacceptable. A one-dimensional concept, for example, is that of "vital" depression. It indicates a syndrome (the syndrome described as endogenous depression in Anglo-American literature). In aetiological terms, however, it is lacking although the "vital" depression is nonspecific in this respect (57, 60). A "vital" endogenous depression may occur not only in response to mainly hereditary factors, but also as a result of intrapsychic tension, pressure exerted by the environment and acquired somatic diseases, or combinations of these factors. In some instances there is no demonstrable cause (ideopathic form). This means that, where possible, the aetiology of a "vital" depression should be indicated. And the same applies to the course, which is likewise variable. There may be a single phase in the course of a lifetime, a recurrent course with complete recovery after each phase, or a recurrent course with incomplete recovery after each phase and transitions to chronic depression. Finally, in the case of a recurrent course, there may be exclusively depressive phases (unipolar depression) or a combination of depressive and manic or hypomanic phases (bipolar depression).

My second example is "personal" depression (73). Like the previous example, I select this because it gives me an opportunity at the same time to elucidate the nomenclature I shall use in this paper. By the term "personal" depression I refer to the *syndrome* described in Anglo-American literature as neurotic or reactive depression. Aetiology and course are not indicated in the term "personal" depression. Psychogenic factors usually play an important aetiological role, but environmental factors are also important, to a varying extent. The significance of heredity is usually minimized in advance, and seldom evaluated; but this is not justifiable (90). The natural history of this sydrome has hardly been systematically studied so far, but it is certainly variable. A neurotic breakdown can occur once in a lifetime or recur frequently, tending towards chronicity in the long run. By this I merely mean to say that a diagnosis of "personal" depression is incomplete, and should be supplemented by data on aetiology and course.

Similarly, a term such as obsessional state indicates a syndrome but by no means its aetiology and course. Compulsive symptoms can be the disastrous end product of an abnormal psychological development; but they can also be observed in depressions, certain types of schizophrenia, and in association with certain morphological brain lesions. The course can be malignant (with resistance to therapy, progressively increasing ritual, and deterioration of the personality structure) or relatively benign (responsive to psychotherapy or to antidepressants).

One-Word Diagnoses

Apart from one- or two-dimensional diagnoses, there is another factor which causes confusion in psychiatric practice: the use of one-word diagnoses. It is evident from the above that these diagnoses are multi-interpretable by definition. Let us take the term schizophrenia. It is suggestive of a nosological entity in the sense used by Kraepelin, as if the term defined fairly accurately the aetiology, symptomatology and prognosis of the disease. Nothing could be less true. There is the most profound confusion about what schizophrenia is and is not. I have discussed this situation elsewhere (74).

Another drawback of a one-word diagnosis is that it can be used in several different ways: sometimes it indicates a particular (psychodynamically interpreted) aetiology; in other cases it indicates a syndrome. Typical examples are such diagnosis as neurosis and hysteria.

In sum, I believe that the consistent use of three-dimensional diagnosis offers the only possibility of finding our way out of the labyrinth of present day confusion.

2. PATHOGENESIS: A FUTURE FOURTH DIMENSION IN PSYCHIATRIC DIAGNOSIS

Apart from the triad of aetiology, symptomatology and prognosis, medicine recognizes a fourth principle of classification: that of pathogenesis. This means classification on the basis of the physical substrate which generates the disease symptoms. In principle, this criterion is valid in psychiatry also (58, 59, 61). In this context I define *pathogenesis* as the complex of cerebral functional disorders which enables psychopathological disturbances to occur. I define *aetiology* as the complex of factors (somatic, psychological and environmental) responsible for the development of these functional disorders.

Recently, there have been suggestions that the pathogenesis is not only valid as a principle in psychiatry, but can be applied in actual fact. For the time being this is true more especially for the group of depressions and, so far as cerebral dysfunctions are concerned, for disorders in central monoamine (MA) metabolism. The data on which this statement is based will be discussed in the following sections of this essay. I shall divide these data into two groups: 1) data which indicate that the central MA metabolism can be disturbed in depressions, and 2) data which indicate that the presence of these disorders probably has consequences for the therapy to be instituted.

3. STUDY OF THE HUMAN CENTRAL MA METABOLISM

Antidepressant medication was introduced in 1958 as a new therapy for depressions. Almost simultaneously, but independently, two different types of compound with an antidepressant effect had been discovered: tricyclic antidepressants (prototype: imipramine, Tofranil) and monoamine oxidase (MAO) inhibitors (prototype: iproniazide, Marsilid). Although tricyclic antidepressants and MAO inhibitors are unrelated in terms of chemical structure, they proved to have two similarities. In psychopathological terms, they exert a beneficial effect on depressions, particularly on a certain syndrome—"vital" depression. In biochemical terms, they behave as MA agonists in the brain, albeit via different mechanisms. MAO inhibitors inhibit the degradation of MA, while tricyclic antidepressants inhibit the (re)uptake of MA into the neuron. Both processes are believed to increase the amount of MA available at the postsynaptic MA receptors.

These findings raised two questions. First, is the therapeutic effect of antidepressants related to their ability to potentiate MA? Second, are those types of depression that usually show a favorable response to these compounds characterized by a functional deficiency in catecholamines (CA) and/or 5-hydroxytryptamine (5-HT; serotonin) in the brain?

The following study addresses the second question. Several strategies have been used: a) postmortem examination of the brains of suicide victims; b) determination of MA metabolites in peripheral body fluids in depressive patients; c) determination, in depressive patients, of the baseline concentrations of MA metabolites in the CSF and their accumulation after administration of probenecid; d) study of the behavioral effects of drugs which either inhibit or stimulate the synthesis of one of the MA.

The second strategy is unreliable. It is unlikely that the overall body metabolism of an MA is correlated with its cerebral metabolism. The only possible exception is the renal excretion of the NA metabolite 3-methoxy-4-hydroxyphenylglycol, which will be discussed in section 4 of this paper.

The probenecid technique is based on the following principle. Probenecid blocks the transport of acid MA metabolites from the CNS to the blood stream. This applies in particular to the transport of 5-hydroxy-

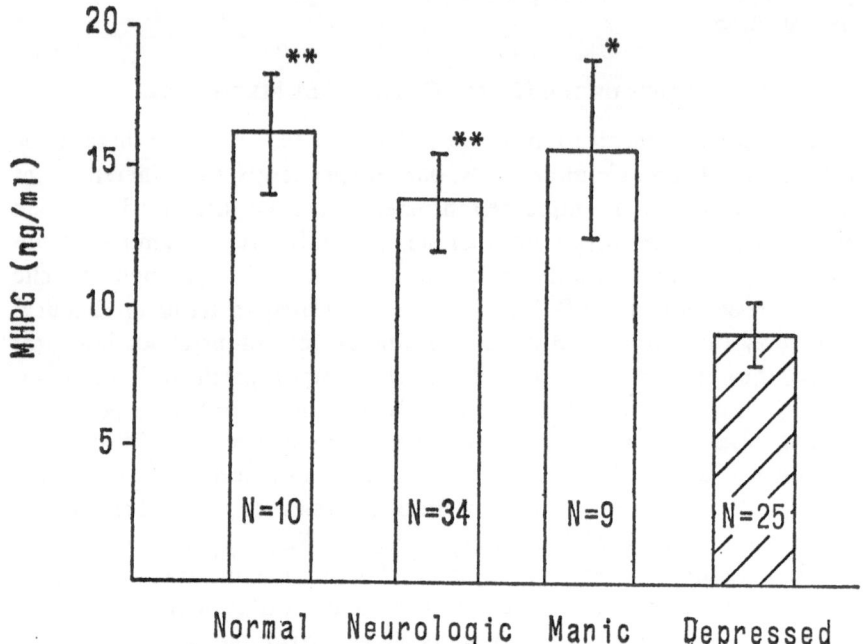

FIGURE 1: Low MHPG concentration in depressed patients. Levels of MHPG in depressed patients were significantly lower than those in other groups (*, P < 0.05; **, P < 0.01; Student's t-test, two-tailed) (56).

indoleacetic acid (5-HIAA) and that of homovanillic acid (HVA)—the principal degradation products of 5-HT and dopamine (DA), respectively. As a result of the transport block, these acids accumulate in the CNS, including the CSF, at a rate which is related to their rate of synthesis. Determination of their accumulation, therefore, supplies an indication of their rate of degradation. The latter is believed to be high when accumulation is high, and low when accumulation is low.

Considered separately, the information obtained by each of these methods is limited. Their limitations and imperfections need not be discussed here; this has been done elsewhere (73, 75). In this context I wish only to state that, when the methods are taken together, they really reveal a pattern which, in my opinion, is meaningful, as the following sections will demonstrate.

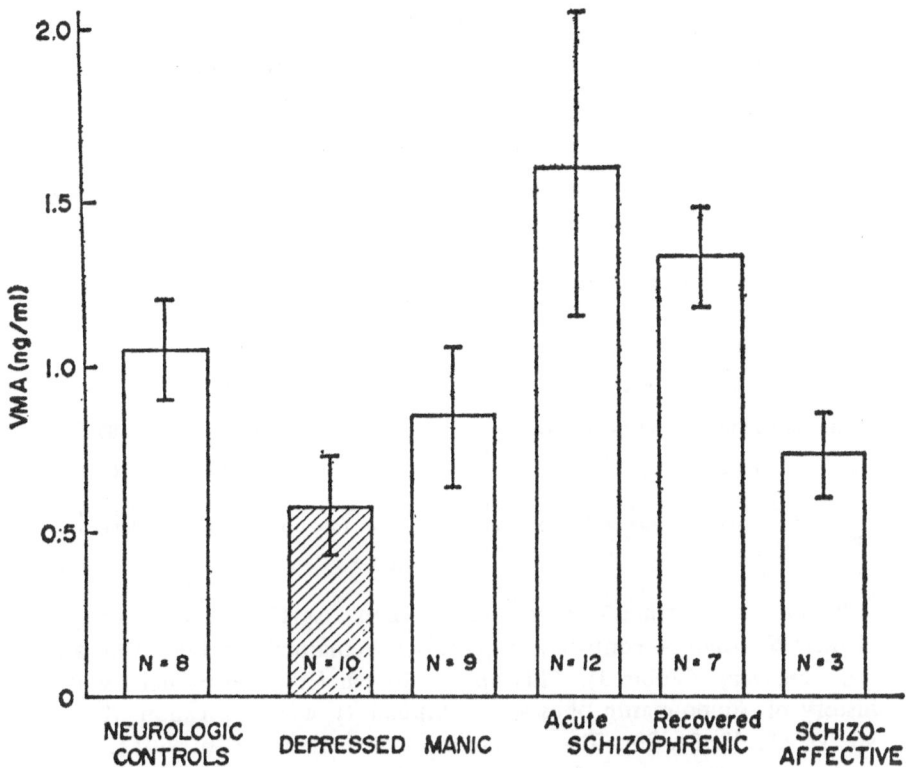

FIGURE 2: Mean (± S.E.) baseline VMA levels in ng/ml in lumbar CSF from different psychiatric groups and neurological controls. Mean VMA for the depressed patients is lower than that for the controls ($P < 0.05$), acute schizophrenics ($P < 0.01$), or recovered schizophrenics ($P < 0.05$) (39).

4. DISORDERS IN CENTRAL NA METABOLISM IN DEPRESSIONS

Chemical Research

Noradrenaline (NA), in the human CNS, is oxidized minimally to vanillylmandelic acid (VMA) and for the most part reduced to 3-methoxy-4-hydroxyphenylglycol (MHPG). Outside the CNS this proportion is reversed. In a series of 25 patients with so-called primary depressions (25), the NIMH group found a decreased concentration of MHPG (Figure 1) and of VMA (Figure 2) in the CSF (39, 56). Shopsin et al. (91) reported normal values, but their group of patients was small ($n = 8$) and heterogeneous.

TABLE 1

Excretion of MHPG in Depressed Patients with Primary and
Secondary Affective Disorder and in a Healthy Control
Group (21)

Group	Number	Excretion of MHPG per 24-hour urine (µg)*	
		Mean	*SEM*
Primary affective disorder patients			
bipolar patients	5	911	154
recurrent unipolar patients	9	1066	86
single-episode unipolar patients	7	1073	140
Undiagnosed affective disorder patients	11	1280	185
Healthy subjects	21	1348	67

* An analysis of variance indicated significant differences between groups, and each of the patient groups differed significantly from the control group (p < 0.05, Duncan's Multiple Range Test).

Patients with primary depressions also had a smaller urinary excretion of MHPG than a control group, which remained smaller even after their recovery (Table 1). This applies in particular to patients with a history of (hypo)manic phases, i.e., bipolar type of depression (21, 36, 46, 47, 48, 83, 84, 89). The phenomenon was observed in patients with motor retardation as well as in agitated patients (21), indicating that the decreased MHPG excretion is not likely to be of peripheral origin, as it is not related to the patient's motor inactivity. Since renal MHPG is regarded as a gross indicator of extraneuronal NA degradation in the CNS (40), the above-mentioned phenomenon might indicate a reduced release of NA in central NA-ergic neurons. The transport of MHPG from the CNS is not probenecid-sensitive. The probenecid technique is therefore unsuitable for a study of central NA metabolism (35, 41).

Postmortem findings have failed to support the hypothesis that NA deficiency plans a role in the pathogenesis of depressions. The concentrations of NA and a few enzymes involved in its synthesis were normal (52).

Pharmacological Research

If NA depletion plays a role in the pathogenesis of certain types of depression, then it may be expected that an exogenously induced NA depletion has a depressant effect, while enhancement of the NA supply in NA-deficient patients should have an antidepressant effect. α-Methyl-p-tyrosine (α-MT) inhibits tyrosine hydroxylase and therefore NA synthesis. In subhuman primates it induced behavior changes reminiscent of depression (77). In humans this has not been unequivocally demonstrated, but the agent has been used on only a limited scale. In manic phases it is therapeutically effective (10).

Of course α-MT inhibits not only the synthesis of NA but also that of DA. Exclusive inhibition of NA synthesis calls for an inhibitor of DA-β-hydroxylase. Fusaric acid is such a compound (53). It aggravates the condition of manic patients (80), rendering human subjects not so much depressive as psychotic. It is not clear whether this is an effect of fusaric acid or a result of the fact that the patient is deprived of effective medication.

Since tyrosine hydroxylase is normally saturated with substrate, administration of tyrosine does not lead to an increase in NA synthesis (43). Dopa stimulates DA production in particular, but little of it is transformed to NA (12). Dihydroxyphenylserine (DOPS), an amino-acid which is not naturally present in the human organism, is directly decarboxylated to NA without intermediate DA synthesis (6). In depressive patients, however, this agent has not been tested.

5. NA Metabolism and Treatment of Depressions

If decreased MHPG concentrations in CSF and urine denote reduced degradation of NA in the brain, and if this reduced degradation is of importance in the pathogenesis of depression, then a therapeutic effect may be expected from enhancement of central NA activity. This expectation would seem to be corroborated by empirical findings, and the postulates preceding this expectation therefore gain plausibility.

Maas et al. (47) found, and Beckmann and Goodwin (4) confirmed, that the therapeutic efficacy of imipramine and desipramine (Pertofran) is greater when pretherapeutic urinary excretion of MHPG is low than when pretherapeutic MHPG excretion is normal or high (Table 2; Figure 3). However, the low MHPG excretors responded to d-amphetamine with improved mood, while the normal excretors showed an unchanged or dysphoric mood (24). These anti-depressant compounds can be assumed capable of relatively selective potentiation of central NA. Thus, imipramine and desipramine have a more marked inhibitory effect

TABLE 2

Relation Between Tricyclic Response and 24-Hour
Urinary MHPG Excretion in Unipolar Patients (4)

| | 24-hour urinary MHPG excretion (mg/24 hr) | | difference* |
	responders	non-responders	
amitryptyline	2.17 ± 0.9	1.21 ± 0.9	p < 0.01
(Tryptisol)	(n = 4)	(n = 4)	
imipramine	1.10 ± 0.7	1.93 ± .13	p < 0.001
(Tofranil)	(n = 9)	(n = 7)	

* student t-test, two-tailed

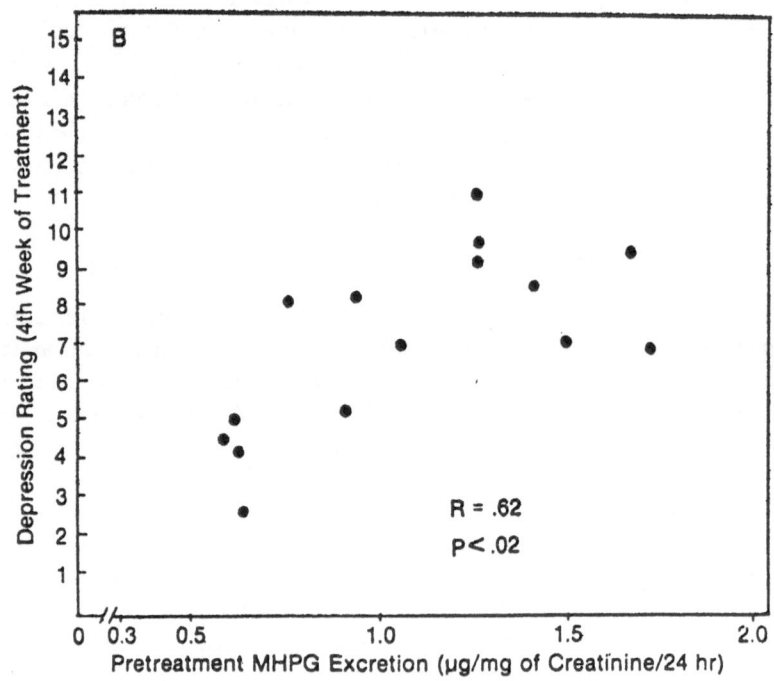

FIGURE 3: Micrograms of MHPG per milligram of creatinine excreted
in urine per 24 hours prior to drug treatment plotted against depression ratings during the fourth week of treatment with imipramine
(47).

on reuptake of NA into the neuron than on reuptake of 5-HT (14, 15). This is more evident for desipramine than for imipramine, but the latter is demethylated to desipramine in the organism. We may therefore assume that these compounds enhance central noradrenergic activity more than they do central serotonergic activity. Amphetamines increase the amount of CA available at the central receptors via different mechanisms (MAO inhibition, inhibition of reuptake and CA release). Their influence on the 5-HT system is only marginal (76).

Depressive patients with a high or normal MHPG excretion show a better response to amitriptyline (Elavil) than patients with a low MHPG excretion (4, 82) (Table 2). Amitriptyline is an antidepressant which inhibits reuptake of 5-HT more markedly than that of NA (44, 79). It is conceivable that less favorable results in low MHPG excretors are based on the relatively slight NA-potentiating effect of amitriptyline, while the favorable effect in normal or high MHPG excretors is based on its relatively marked influence on 5-HT. The second part of this hypothesis would become plausible only if it could be demonstrated that a central 5-HT deficiency probably existed before treatment in the patients showing the favorable response. Pertinent studies have not yet been made. Nor have any studies been devoted to the question whether variations in renal MHPG excretion in these patients are reflected in the MHPG concentration in the CSF.

As imipramine is demethylated in the organism to desipramine, so also is amitriptyline demethylated to nortriptyline (Aventyl). As pointed out, amitriptyline exerts no marked influence on NA uptake, but nortriptyline does (37, 97). This fact does not automatically devalue the above-mentioned hypothesis, for it is quite possible that transformation of amitriptyline to the secondary amine is slower than its inactivation, so that no effective concentration of nortriptyline can be built up (48).

The above data warrant the following *conclusions*:

1. Disorders of central NA metabolism which may present in certain categories of depression probably play a role in the pathogenesis of these syndromes. This conclusion is based on two observations: a) depressive patients showing indications of a central NA deficiency have a more favorable response to NA-potentiating antidepressants than depressive patients with no indications of such deficiency; b) the former group shows a less favorable response to antidepressants with relatively little NA-potentiating capacity than the latter group.

2. Disorders of NA metabolism are not characteristic of depression in general but only of certain categories of depression.
3. Renal MHPG excretion supplies information which is of importance in determining indications for antidepressant medication.

6. DISORDERS OF CENTRAL DA METABOLISM IN DEPRESSIONS

Chemical Research

In rats, HVA and 3,4-dihydroxyphenylacetic acid (DOPAC) are the principal degradation products of DA. In the human, DA is largely converted to HVA. DOPAC is found in only very small quantities in the human CSF even after administering l-dopa for short or long periods. (102). HVA largely originates from the brain in lumbar CSF as the spinal cord contains hardly any DA. The largest contribution is probably made by the nigrostriatal DA system (29).

Several investigators have reported a decreased HVA concentration in the CSF in depressions (8, 50, 54, 78), although the finding was not always statistically significant (64, 101). Moreover, the probenecid-induced HVA accumulation in the CSF was decreased, and this is also indicative of a decreased central DA turnover (33, 64, 66, 78, 94). An additional argument in favor of a disturbed DA turnover was supplied by Sjöström and Roos (94), who administered methylperidol as well as probenecid to a number of test subjects. Methylperidol is a neuroleptic of the butyrophenone series, which greatly stimulates the DA turnover in the brain, probably secondarily to postsynaptic DA receptor block. Given an undisturbed DA production, this compound can be expected to cause a marked increase of the probenecid-induced HVA accumulation in the CSF. This was observed by these workers, except in the depressive group where the augmented increase caused by methylperidol was much less marked.

According to Goodwin and Post (33), a disorder of DA metabolism is most marked in "vital" endogenous depressions with a unipolar course. We ourselves found that the decreased HVA accumulation is not characteristic of "vital" depression but a phenomenon related to the state of motor retardation (64, 66, 71) (Table 3). Since motor retardation is much more common in "vital" than in "personal" (neurotic) depressions, the disorder of DA metabolism *seems* to be a characteristic of "vital" depression. However, the phenomenon is also observed in "personal" depressions in which motor retardation is a prominent feature (65). Post-

TABLE 3

Concentration of HVA in CSF in Depressive Patients and
Controls Before and After Probenecid Administration
(in ng-/ml) (64)

	no. of test subjects	before probenecid	after probenecid	difference
depression (retarded and non-retarded)	20	39 ± 16 (14 — 67)	82 ± 43 (27 — 185)	44 ± 38 (0.0 — 130)
retarded depression	8	32 ± 8 (20 — 46)	53 ± 32 (27 — 114)	20 ± 28 (0.0 — 74)
non-retarded depression	12	43 ± 17 (14 — 67)	106 ± 36 (40 — 185)	63 ± 37 (10 — 130)
control	12	42 ± 16 (21 — 73)	91 ± 26 (59 — 151)	50 ± 33 (23 — 122)

Results are given as means plus or minus s.d. (with range)

mortem studies have failed to reveal any abnormalities in DA metabolism (52).

Pharmacological Research

The effect of inhibition of CA synthesis on behavior has been discussed in Section 4, and the effect of increased DA synthesis is discussed in Section 7.

7. DA METABOLISM AND TREATMENT OF DEPRESSIONS

In the CNS exogenous l-dopa is for the most part converted to DA, but a small amount is converted to NA. Its therapeutic effect in a psychopathologically and biochemically undifferentiated group of depressions is unspectacular, particularly if evaluated on the basis of differences in total scores, disregarding changes in certain components of the depressive syndrome (32, 49). Different findings are obtained when biochemical variables are considered in the test arrangement and profiles rather than when total scores are compared.

Ten depressive patients were selected on the basis of a biochemical criterion: the response to probenecid of HVA in the CSF (68). In 5

TABLE 4

DA Metabolism Before Treatment and Response to L-Dopa
in Depression (68)

	no. of patients	HVA accumulation* (ng/ml)	Motor retardation* before treatment	after treatment
DA-deficient patients	5	74 (65 — 90)	6.8 (4 — 8)	2.7 (0 — 3)
non-DA-deficient patients	5	121 (107 — 143)	2.1 (0 — 3)	2.4 (0 — 3)

* Group mean and range

patients it was more, and in 5 it was less than 100 ng/ml. Motor retardation, measured by two independent raters using a 10-point scale, was more marked in the second than in the first group. Mood scores in the two groups were not significantly different. All patients were treated with l-dopa and a peripheral decarboxylase inhibitor for two weeks. At the end of this period, motor retardation had virtually disappeared in the patients with a low HVA response (Table 4), while in patients with a normal response the motor status remained unchanged. This was to be expected because in this group pre-therapeutic motor activity had been hardly abnormal. The mood scores were not significantly influenced by l-dopa. In both groups, finally, the HVA response to probenecid during treatment was about twice the pre-therapeutic response. The low responders too, were evidently able to convert l-dopa to DA. In practical terms, l-dopa is not a useful antidepressant because its influence on mood is too slight. Moreover, the activating effect of l-dopa in depressions is not superior to that of tricyclic antidepressants with an activating component.

In a second experiment, clomipramine (Anafranil) was compared with nomifensine in a double-blind study of a group of patients with "vital" depressions. Nomifensine is a compound with a relatively selective stimulating effect on postsynaptic DA repectors. It was significantly more effective in patients with a subnormal than in those with a normal HVA response to probenecid before treatment. In the clomipramine group this difference was not observed (Van Scheijen and Van Praag, to be published).

My *conclusion* from these data is a dual one:

1. Since dopa has a favorable effect on certain (motor) components of the depressive syndrome in DA-deficient patients, and fails to produce this effect in patients with a normal DA metabolism, I regard it as plausible that the biochemical disorder plays a role in the pathogenesis of these components;

2. The current antidepressants, i.e., roughly speaking the so-called tricyclic and tetracyclic antidepressants, exert only a slight influence on central DA metabolism, and consequently identification of a central DA deficiency in depressive patients can have implications for the treatment to be instituted.

8. Disorders of Central 5-HT Metabolism in Depressions

CSF Studies

The principal degradation product of the central 5-HT metabolism is 5-hydroxyindoleacetic acid (5-HIAA). This applies to human and animal subjects alike (87). The human CSF contains only traces of the corresponding alcohol, 5-hydroxytryptophol (102). Part of the 5-HIAA found in lumbar CSF is of spinal origin, and another part originates from higher levels (29).

Data on the baseline concentration of 5-HIAA in CSF are not unequivocal. Decreased values have been reported (3, 19, 50), but there have also been reports on normal values (e.g., 78, 101). However, since the psychopathological classification of the syndromes studied was often rather imperfect, it is conceivable that characteristics inherent in certain subcategories were overlooked. Asberg et al. (2) demonstrated that this is a real possibility. Within a group of patients with endogenous depressions, some showed a normal and others a decreased 5-HIAA concentration in the CSF. The 5-HIAA concentrations measured by means of gas chromatography/mass spectrometry showed a bimodal distribution. This suggests that the group of endogenous depressions, although tending towards homogeneity in terms of symptomatology, is a heterogeneous group in biochemical terms, i.e., in terms of pathogenesis. A few years earlier van Praag and Korf (63) had reached a similar conclusion on the basis of results of the probenecid test. Within a group of patients with "vital" depressions, the 5-HIAA response to probenecid was decreased in about 40% of patients (Figure 4). On the basis of this finding they postulated the biochemical heterogeneity of the group of "vital" depressions; this group was believed to include forms with and without demonstrable central 5-HT deficiency.

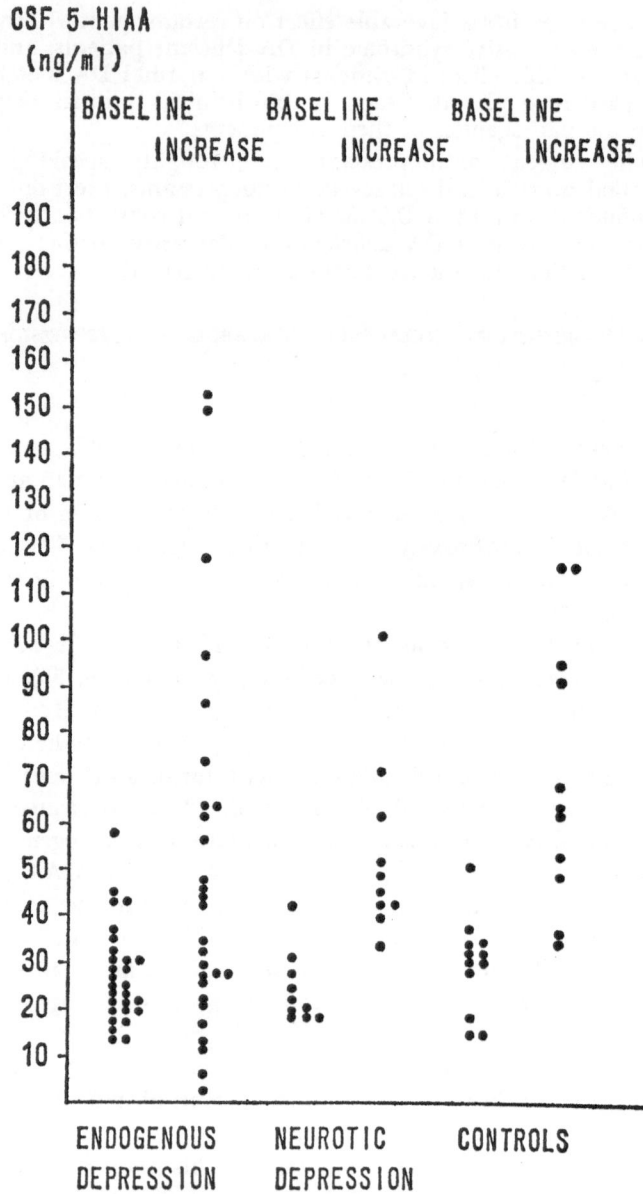

FIGURE 4. Baseline 5-HIAA concentration in CSF and increase of concentration after probenecid in endogenous (vital) depressions, neurotic depressions and controls (66).

The decreased 5-HIAA accumulation in "vital" depressions has been confirmed by several groups of investigators (34, 78, 94). Only Bowers (9) reported normal values, but this may have been due to the heterogeneity of the group of patients studied. However, the group of "personal" depressions shows virtually no instances of decreased 5-HIAA accumulation (66).

Postmortem Studies

The results of postmortem studies in suicide victims are not unequivocal but do point in the same direction: a tendency of the 5-HT and 5-HIAA concentrations to decrease in the brain, especially in the raphe nuclei. The raphe nuclei are the site of predilection of 5-HT in the brain (7, 45, 55, 88) (Table 5). This phenomenon might indicate that 5-HT synthesis was decreased prior to death. The different results reported by different investigators can possibly be explained on the basis of the fact that the histories of these suicide victims were not always known; moreover, suicide is also committed by patients other than those with pathological depressions.

Pharmacological Research

Human central serotonergic activity can be suppressed by two different ways: with the aid of p-chlorophenylalanine (pcpa), an inhibitor of tryptophan hydroxylase, and with the aid of methysergide (Deseril), a 5-HT antagonist. In this context it is to be noted that, although this is often assumed, it is not certain that reduction of 5-HT synthesis causes decreased serotonergic function. Depressions have not been described after these two compounds (23, 26). On the other hand, pcpa abolishes the therapeutic effect of imipramine (Tofranil) within a few days (93). It can therefore not be stated that suppression of serotonergic activity brought about by pharmacological means has no effect on mood regulation.

The possibilities of relatively selective stimulation of human central 5-HT activity are limited. The 5-HT precursors tryptophan and 5-hydroxytryptophan (5-HTP) increase 5-HT synthesis, as demonstrated by the increased 5-HIAA accumulation in response to probenecid (33, 70). The effect of 5-HTP is shown in Table 6. The effects of tryptophan and 5-HTP in depressions are discussed in Section 9. The influence of chloramphetamines on central 5-HT is a fairly selective but complex

TABLE 5

Concentrations of 5-HIAA and 5-HT in the Raphe Nuclei of
Controls and Suicides (45)

5-HIAA (µg/g)

Raphe nuclei	Controls Mean ± SEM	n	Suicides Mean ± SEM	n
Centralis superior	12.37 ± 0.65 (11.25 — 14.53)	5	12.39 ± 0.91 (9.19 — 14.61)	5
Dorsalis	7.04 ± 0.59 (5.85 — 8.63)	5	6.14 — 0.52 (5.00 — 7.79)	5
Pontis	7.66 ± 0.57 (6.21 — 8.92)	5	7.12 ± 0.68 (5.42 — 9.55)	5
Centralis inferior	4.49 ± 0.43 (3.63 — 5.77)	5	4.01 ± 0.32 (3.14 — 4.67)	5
Obscurus	2.86 ± 0.24 (2.00 — 3.46)	5	3.36 ± 0.31 (2.46 — 4.24)	5
Pallidus	2.28 ± 0.16 (1.85 — 2.67)	5	2.25 ± 0.20 (1.90 — 2.74)	4

5-HT (µg/g)

Raphe nuclei	Controls Mean ± SEM	n	Suicides Mean ± SEM	n
Centralis superior	2.25 ± 0.19 (1.88 — 2.97)	5	1.86 ± 0.16 (1.41 — 2.26)	5
Dorsalis	2.22 ± 0.13 (1.92 — 2.56)	5	1.55 ± 0.12[a] (1.23 — 1.90)	5
Pontis	1.34 ± 0.21 (0.80 — 1.89)	5	1.04 ± 0.13 (0.65 — 1.38)	5
Centralis inferior	1.32 ± 0.12 (0.94 — 1.47)	5	0.95 ± 0.07[b] (0.69 — 1.09)	5
Obscurus	1.07 ± 0.14 (0.62 — 1.39)	5	1.02 ± 0.14 (0.75 — .56)	5
Pallidus	0.61 ± 0.09 (0.44 — 0.91)	5	0.42 ± 0.12 (0.28 — 0.76)	4

n is the number of brains examined. Ranges are given in parentheses. Significantly different from controls: [a] $p < 0.01$; [b] $p < 0.05$.

TABLE 6

5-HIAA Accumulation in CSF After Probenecid Before Treatment
and During Treatment with 1-5-HTP (200 mg per Day) in
Combination with a Peripheral Decarboxylase Inhibitor
(MK 486 150 mg per day) (70)

	no. of patients	CSF 5-HIAA after probenecid (ng/ml) before treatment	after treatment	CSF probenecid µg/ml
low 5-HIAA response	5	26 ± 11.1	63 ± 22.5	8.7 ± 1.9
normal 5-HIAA response	5	90 ± 32.3	150 ± 40.8	9.80 ± 3.0

one, which comprises at least four components: 1) inhibition of 5-HT synthesis; 2) release of 5-HT from the synaptic vesicles; 3) inhibition of 5-HT reuptake; and 4) MAO inhibition. At least in acute experiments, the net effect is reported to be enhancement of central 5-HT activity (27). When used in depressive patients, they produce a therapeutic effect which differs from that of the non-chlorinated amphetamine derivatives, and closely resembles that of the conventional antidepressants (67, 72).

9. 5-HT METABOLISM AND TREATMENT OF DEPRESSIONS

Hypotheses

Assuming that: a) a low 5-HIAA response to probenecid indeed indicates a diminished 5-HT turnover in the brain, and b) the suspected 5-HT deficiency plays a role in the pathogenesis of (certain components) of the "vital" depression, the following hypotheses seem justifiable.

1. 5-HT-potentiating antidepressants will be therapeutically effective in "5-HT-deficient depressions" but not, or in a lesser degree, in depressive patients without a demonstrable central 5-HT deficiency.
2. Antidepressants with a mainly NA-potentiating effect will produce little effect in "5-HT-deficient depressions."

Precursor Studies

The 5-HT precursors tryptophan and 5-HTP stimulate central 5-HT synthesis in test animals. That they do the same in human individuals is

TABLE 7

Increase of CSF 5-HIAA in Response to Probenecid Before Treatment
and Effectiveness of 1-5-HTP (65)

| | CSF 5-HIAA level (ng/ml) | | | CSF probenecid level (μg/ml) |
	before probenecid	after probenecid	increase	
5-HTP, improved*	18 (16-22)	35 (28-48)	16 (11-26)	7.2 (5.0-10.7)
5-HTP, not improved*	17 (13-22)	71 (61-81)	50 (39-68)	6.5 (5.5-7.5)
placebo**	25 ± 9 (13-33)	72 ± 33 (51-129)	47 ± 39 (20-116)	12.6 ± 6.2 (4.0-19.0)
non-depressive** control group	32 ± 14 (21-66)	112 ± 46 (60-179)	80 ± 49 (26-153)	9.1 ± 3.5 (3.0-16.5)

* group mean and range
** group mean with standard deviation and range

apparent from the increased 5-HIAA response to probenecid which they produce (22, 70). It has been demonstrated that low 5-HIAA responders, too, are capable of converting 5-HTP to 5-HT (70).

The antidepressant activity of l-tryptophan is controversial; some authors described it as effective (18, 38), while others regarded it as no better than a placebo (16, 51). So far, however, clinical studies have not been related to data on the central 5-HT metabolism. It remains possible, therefore, that a 5-HT-deficient subgroup exists which is susceptible to tryptophan. This could explain the variability of results reported so far (62). The observation that a combination of an MAO inhibitor with tryptophan is more effective than an MAO inhibitor alone, has not been contradicted so far (17, 31).

The still scanty research so far done with 5-HTP indicates that my plea in favor of considering biochemical data in the interpretation of therapeutic results obtained with new, potential antidepressants, has not been groundless. For van Praag et al. (65) found that 1-5-HTP can be therapeutically effective in depressions and that this effect occurs in particular in low 5-HIAA responders to probenecid (Table 7). Good results obtained with 5-HTP have also been reported by Sano (81) and Takahashi et al. (95). However, theirs were open studies. In a small, biochemically unclassified group of 6 depressive patients, Brodie et al. (11) were unsuccessful with 5-HTP. That the 5-HTP effect in depressions is not a non-specific one but is really produced via 5-HT is probable in view of the fact that the 5-HTP effect is potentiated by the relatively selective 5-HT reuptake inhibitor clomipramine (Anafranil) in doses which are not effective (69). However, a "mirror" experiment concerning the question whether a relatively selective NA reuptake inhibitor such as nortriptyline lacks this effect of clomipramine, has not been carried out. The combination of l-tryptophan and clomipramine has also been reported to produce a more marked antidepressant effect than clomipramine alone (98). In normal test subjects, too, a positive effect of l-5-HTP on the mood level has been reported (96).

There is as yet no certainty about the value or lack of value of 5-HT precursors in depressions. I consider it to be of essential importance that future studies account for the patient's pre-therapeutic biochemical status.

CSF 5-HIAA and Nortriptyline

Åsberg et al. (1) studied the question whether there is a relation between the 5-HIAA concentration in CSF and the therapeutic response to nortriptyline. They found that the therapeutic effect of nortriptyline was less pronounced in depressive patients with a CSF 5-HIAA concentration of less than 15 ng/ml than in patients with higher 5-HIAA concentrations (Table 8). The plasma nortriptyline concentration was within the therapeutic range in both groups.

Nortriptyline is a relatively selective inhibitor of the "NA pump" (14, 15). It seems a plausible hypothesis that the group with low 5-HIAA shows little response because nortriptyline potentiates chiefly NA. In that case it might be expected that such patients would benefit more from an antidepressant which chiefly potentiates 5 HT, e.g., clomipramine. Research into this hypothesis is now in progress (see next section).

CSF 5-HIAA and Clomipramine

In 30 patients with "vital" (endogenous) depressions van Praag and co-workers studied the relation between probenecid-induced 5-HIAA accumulation (interpreted as an indicator of central 5-HT turnover) prior to medication and the therapeutic effect of clomipramine, a mainly 5-HT-potentiating antidepressant. The diagnosis was unipolar depression in 16 patients and bipolar in 7, while the remaining patients were in

TABLE 8

Relation Between Pre-therapeutic CSF 5-HIAA and Clinical Improvement During Nortriptyline Medication (150 mg Per Day), as Measured with the Aid of Cronholm-Ottosson Scale in 20 Patients Suffering from Vital ("Endogenous") Depressions (1)

5-HIAA in CSF (ng/ml)	number of patients	severity of depression (rating score)		amelioration (reduction in rating score) mean ± S.D.
		before treatment, mean ± S.D.	during treatment, mean ± S.D.	
6.0 — 14.6	7	14.0 ± 3.1*	10.0 ± 8.3	4.0 ± 7.7**
17.7 — 37.5	13	11.7 ± 3.1*	3.9 ± 3.1	7.8 ± 2.8***

* t to compare means = 1.55 (N.S.)
** does not differ significantly from zero; t = 1.38
*** significantly different from zero; t = 10.26, p < 0.001

TABLE 9

5-HT Metabolism/Outcome Clomipramine Treatment

1. 30 Patients with depression. F:18, M:12. Age 19-65 (Av. 44)

2. Syndrome: vital depression

3. Course: Unipolar 16, Bipolar 7, First episode 7

4. Aetiology: Hereditary factors   = 18

   Psychogenic/environmental factors   = 21

   Acquired somatic factors   = 3

   Unknown   = 5

5. Medication: 225 mg Clomipramine per day for 3 weeks

their first depressive phase (Table 9). The drug was administered for 3 weeks at a daily dosage of 225 mg. The therapeutic effect of medication increased by as much as pre-therapeutic 5-HIAA accumulation had been lower (Figure 5), suggesting a negative correlation between the two variables.

After 3 weeks, 8 patients were considered not to have improved at all. Clomipramine was discontinued in these cases and replaced by a placebo for one week. The placebo period was followed by 3 weeks of daily administration of 150 mg nortriptyline, a mainly NA-potentiating antidepressant. Placebo and nortriptyline were given in capsules identical to those in which clomipramine had been administered. Neither raters nor patients were aware of the switch to placebo and then to nortriptyline. Of these 8 patients, 5 were considered to have markedly improved at the end of the third week of nortriptyline medication (Table 10). No correlation was found between pre-therapeutic CSF MHPG concentration and therapeutic effect of medication (Figure 6). Urinal MHPG excretion was not measured.

Conclusions

The above data warrant the following conclusions:

1. The disorders of central 5-HT metabolism which have been observed in certain depressive syndromes are not a secondary phenomenon but probably play a role in the pathogenesis of

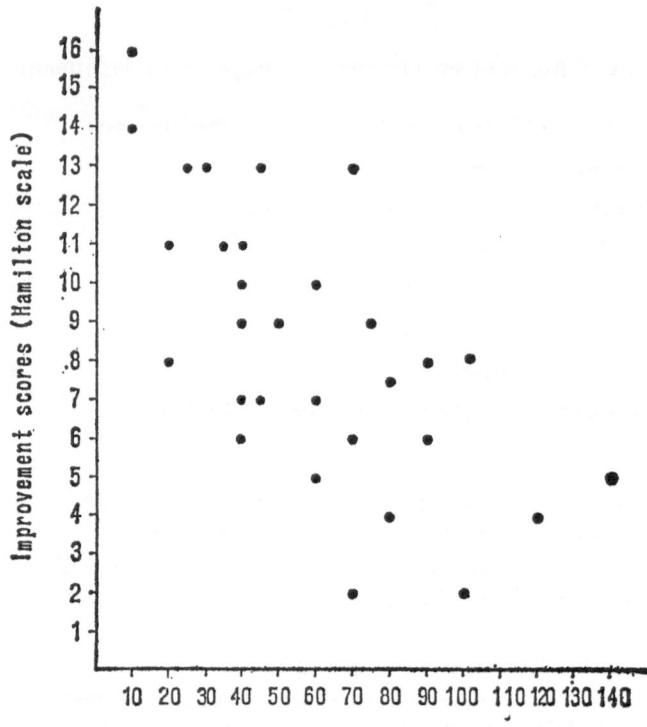

CSF 5-HIAA accumulation after probenecid (ng/ml)

FIGURE 5: Relation between pre-therapeutic 5-HIAA response to probenecid and clinical improvement during clomipramine medication (225 mg daily) as measured with the aid of the Hamilton scale in 30 patients with vital ("endogenous") depressions. Bravais-Pearson correlation coefficient $r = -0.40$, $p < 0.05$.

these depressions. This conclusion is based on the following data: a) "5-HT-deficient depressions" improve in response to compounds considered to increase the amount of 5-HT available in the brain; their therapeutic effect is more pronounced than that in patients without a demonstrable central 5-HT deficiency. b) In "5-HT-deficient depressions" the therapeutic effect of an antidepressant with a mostly NA-potentiating effect (e.g., nortriptyline) is less marked than that in patients without a demonstrable defect in central 5-HT metabolism. It is logical to expect these nortriptyline-susceptible patients to be NA-deficient. However, CSF studies have failed to corroborate this expectation. Renal MHPG excre-

TABLE 10

Pre-therapeutic CSF MHPG Concentration and Effect of
Nortriptyline Medication (3 × 50 mg Daily) in 8
Clomipramine-Resistant Depressive Patients

patient	CSF MHPG before treatment (ng/ml)	improvement score after 3 weeks (Hamilton scale)	clearly improved
1	6.5	0	no
2	7.6	+ 5	no
3	8.2	+10	no
4	8.9	+ 2	yes
5	9.8	+16	yes
6	10.1	+11	yes
7	14.7	+17	yes
8	15.9	+13	yes

tion was not determined in these patients. The finding of a decreased excretion would elegantly clinch the hypothesis.

2. Disorders of 5-HT metabolism are characteristic, not of depressions in general but of certain types of "vital" (endogenous) depression.

3. Determination of the CSF 5-HIAA concentration (preferably after probenecid administration) supplies data which can be of significance in the choice of an optimal antidepressant.

10. MA METABOLISM AND TREATMENT OF DEPRESSIONS: GENERAL CONCLUSIONS

I believe that the above discussed relations between MA metabolism and treatment results with compounds which influence MA lend support to two concepts—the concept that disorders of central MA metabolism can play a role in the pathogenesis of "vital" (endogenous) depressions, and the concept that the group of "vital" depressions is a heterogeneous one in biochemical terms. At least two types of "vital" depression exist; 5-HT deficiency plays a role in the pathogenesis of one, while NA deficiency is important in the pathogenesis of the other. Both of these types of depression are indistinguishable in psychopathological terms.

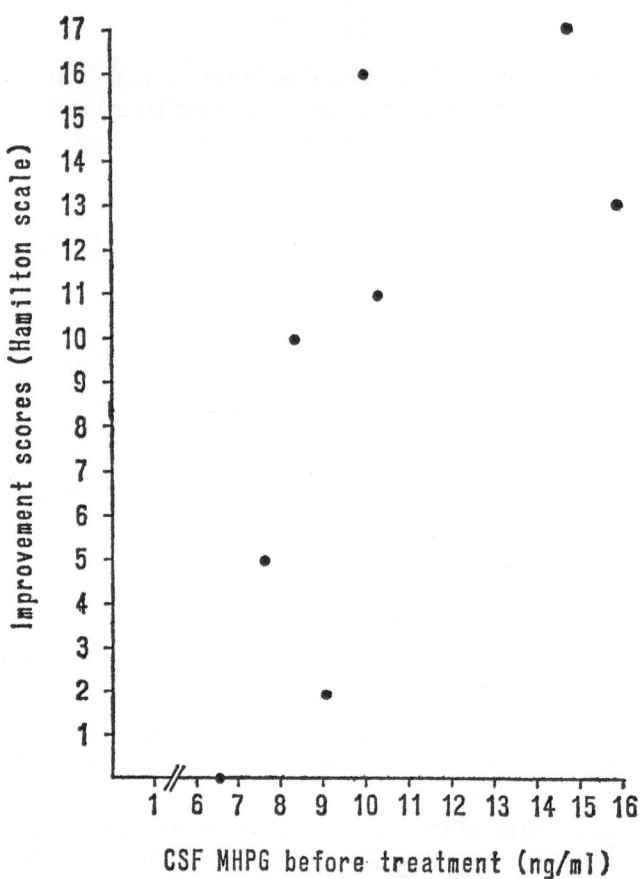

FIGURE 6: Relation between pre-therapeutic CSF MHPG concentration and clinical improvement during nortriptyline medication (150 mg daily), as measured with the aid of the Hamilton scale in 8 patients with vital ("endogenous") depressions and refractory to clomipramine.

Patients of the first group seem to respond best to antidepressants with a strong ability to potentiate 5-HT and less to NA-potentiating compounds, while the reverse applies to the NA-deficient patient. The CSF supplies no reliable information on the presence or absence of a central NA deficiency; according to Maas (48), renal MHPG excretion is more instructive in this respect (cf. Section 5). It was already known that renal MHPG and CSF show a poor correlation (92). A possible explanation is that MHPG in the lumbar CSF is chiefly of spinal, not of cerebral origin (29).

This conclusion raises three new questions.

1. What exactly is the relation between renal MHPG and MHPG in CSF?
2. Can both 5-HT and NA metabolism be disturbed in the same patient, or are "vital" depressions either chiefly 5-HT NA-deficient?
3. What is the therapeutic efficacy of various chemical types of antidepressant in patients with "vital" depressions who show no demonstrable disorders of central MA metabolism?

It is to these questions that answers must be found.

11. SPECIFIC CHEMOPROPHYLAXIS

Let us assume that: 1) the reported disorders of MA metabolism are an expression of a central MA deficiency, and 2) this deficiency contributes to the development of the depressive syndrome. This assumption raises the question whether this deficiency is causal or is merely a predisposing factor, i.e., a factor which increases the risk that a balance of mood will change in a negative direction under certain less favorable circumstances. Longitudinal studies of the biochemical disorders can provide an answer to this question. If the biochemical disorders gradually disappear with the psychopathological disturbances, then this argues in favor of their causal significance; if they persist after abatement of the depression, then they are more likely to be a predisposing factor.

Few longitudinal studies have so far been done. Their results thus far can be summarized as follows. The subnormal HVA response to probenecid returns to normal after normalization of motor activity (70, 73). The decreased urinary MHPG concentration is likewise syndrome-dependent: the phenomenon disappears as the depression disappears (20, 21). No data are available on MHPG in CSF.

The data on 5-HIAA accumulation in response to probenecid point in a different direction. In slightly less than 50% of patients with a low pre-therapeutic 5-HIAA response, the response returns to normal after clinical recovery. In the remaining patients the 5-HIAA response does not increase, or not to normal values. The second probenecid test was

TABLE 11

Prophylactic Action of L-5-HTP in Unipolar and
Bipolar Depression

Patients	: 5; female 3, male 2
Age	: 35-55
Syndrome	: vital (= endogenous) depression
Etiology	: hereditary and psychogenic factors
Course	: bipolar 3, unipolar 2
Pathogenesis	: subnormal 5-HT turnover
Relapse rate	: 3 or more depressive phases in the past 10-14 months

carried out after the patient had been free of symptoms for six months, and without medication for at least one month (73).

If a persistently decreased 5-HIAA accumulation is indeed a factor predisposing to depressions, then chronic administration of 5-HT precursors might have a prophylactic effect. We studied the prophylactic value of 5-HTP in 5 patients suffering from recurrent "vital" depressions with a) a high rate of recurrence, and b) a low 5-HIAA response to probenecid during the depressive phase and after clinical recovery (Table 11). The depression was of the bipolar type in 3 and of the unipolar type in 2 of these patients. They were successfully treated with tricyclic antidepressants and, one month after discontinuation of this treatment, daily administration of 200 mg 1-5-HTP and 100 mg of a peripheral decarboxylase inhibitor (MK 486) was started. After a month the 5-HIAA response to probenecid was found to be quite above normal, demonstrating their ability to convert 5-HTP to 5-HT. No recurrences have so far been observed during a follow-up of one year (Figure 7). In view of these patients' histories this is a striking result, but it is still to be verified by insertion of placebo periods.

I *conclude* that, at least in a number of patients, the decreased 5-HT turnover seems to have the characteristics of a predisposing factor. It might be the biological expression, so to speak, of the increased tendency of some individuals to respond to threatening endogenous or exogenous stimuli by a pathological deterioration of mood.

12. FOUR-DIMENSIONAL PSYCHIATRIC DIAGNOSIS
AND SOME OF ITS CONSEQUENCES

The principal conclusion which I have drawn from the data discussed is that disorders of central MA metabolism can play a role in the patho-

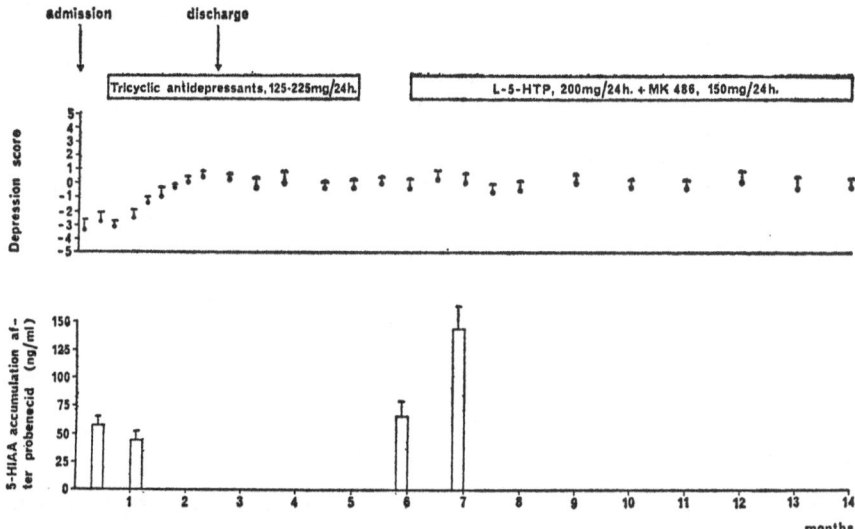

FIGURE 7: Depression scores and 5-HIAA accumulation in response to probenecid in 5 depressive patients during therapeutic administration of a tricyclic antidepressant and prophylactic administration of 1-5-HTP combined with a peripheral decarboxylase inhibitor.

genesis of depressions. If correct, this conclusion would add a fourth criterion or a fourth dimension to the three criteria already applied in the diagnosis of depression: symptomatology, aetiology and course. This fourth criterion would be pathogenesis, in the sense I have conceptualized it previously in Section 2. This observation is important for several reasons.

1. In my opinion it heralds the approach of an era in which biochemical variables will come to play a role in the diagnosis and treatment of psychiatric disorders; an era in which physical examination of the psychiatric patient will not be confined to general neurological and medical screening.

2. Today, the training program of future psychiatrists is still only too often dominated by psychological and sociological approaches. If the above expectation is justified, then equal attention will have to be focused on discussions of the biological determinants of disturbed human behavior. The subject "biological psychiatry" in the curriculum will then have to comprise more than the

knowledge gained from a few talks on prescribing psychotropic drugs.

3. The prototypes of the current psychotropic drugs were all discovered by accident. Their derivatives are not products of purposeful research but result from random variations on existing basic structures. If the above discussed metabolic disorders should indeed prove to be of pathogenetic significance, then they might guide the development of new psychotropic drugs. There are unmistakable indications that this change has already begun. For example, the development of selective 5-HT reuptake inhibitors (e.g., 13, 27) would not have been undertaken without the theory that a central 5-HT deficiency can play a role in the pathogenesis of depression—a theory based on clinical studies. This means that psychopharmacology has entered a new phase in its development.

13. SUMMARY

So far, three criteria have been available for classification of psychiatric syndromes: symptomatology, aetiology and course. Many diagnoses are being made which do not account for each of these three criteria. One-dimensional or two-dimensional diagnoses, however, can be justified only if the characterization of one or two criteria establishes the nature of the other criterion or criteria to a high degree of probability. But this is not the case, and one-dimensional or two-dimensional "diagnoses" therefore make psychiatry unnecessarily opaque.

Medicine recognizes a fourth principle of classification: that based on pathogenesis, i.e., the pathological substrate underlying the disease symptoms. This principle can be applied in psychiatry also. I define the pathogenesis of behavior disorders as the complex of cerebral functional disorders which creates the instrumental conditions for the development of behavior disorders. While until recently this was merely a theoretical possibility, there are now indications that this principle of classification can be made operational in psychiatry also. As regards disturbed behavior, this applies in particular to the group of the depressions, and as regards the cerebral substrate it applies to MA metabolism.

A survey is presented of disorders of central MA metabolism observed in depressions, and of their diagnostic and therapeutic significance. It is concluded that there are two subtypes of "vital" (endogenous) depression: a 5-HT-deficient and a NA-deficient subtype. These subtypes cannot be differentiated in psychopathological terms. The distinction is not an "academic" one, but has its consequences for the treatment to be instituted.

It seems likely that this development will not be confined to the depressions and that, in addition to psychological and environmental factors, biological determinants of disturbed behavior will come to play a role in diagnosis in other psychiatric fields as well. I have no doubt that the reliability and validity of psychiatric diagnoses will increase as a result.

REFERENCES

1. Åsberg, M., Bertilsson, L., Tuck, D., Cronholm, B., & Sjöqvist, F. Indoleamine metabolites in the cerebrospinal fluid of depressed patients before and during treatment with nortriptyline. *Clin. Pharmacol. Ther.*, 14, 277-286, 1972.
2. Åsberg, M., Thorén, P., Träskman, L., Bertilsson, L., & Ringberger, V. Serotonin depression—a biochemical subgroup within the affective disorders? *Science*, 191, 478-480, 1976.
3. Ashcroft, G. W., Crawford, T. B. B., Eccleston, D., Sharman, D. F., McDougall, E. J., Stanton, J. B., & Binns, J. K. 5-Hydroxyindole compounds in the cerebrospinal fluid of patients with psychiatric or neurological diseases. *Lancet*, 2, 1049-1052, 1966.
4. Beckmann, H., & Goodwin, F. K. Antidepressant response to tricyclics and urinary MHPG in unipolar patients. *Archives of General Psychiatry*, 32, 17-21, 1975.
5. Bertilsson, L., Åsberg, M., & Thorén, P. Differential effect of chlorimipramine and nortriptyline on metabolites of serotonin and noradrenaline in the cerebrospinal fluid of depressed patients. *European Journal of Clinical Pharmacology*, 7, 365-368, 1974.
6. Blaschko, H., Burn, J. H., & Langemann, H. The formation of noradrenaline from dihydroxyphenylserine. *British Journal of Pharmacology*, 5, 431-437, 1950.
7. Bourne, H. R., Bunney, W. E., Jr., Colburn, R. W., Davis, J. M., Davis, J. N., Shaw, D. M., & Coppen A. J. Noradrenaline, 5-hydroxytryptamine and 5-hydroxyindoleacetic acid in hindbrain of suicidal patients. *Lancet*, 2, 805-808, 1968.
8. Bowers, M. B., Jr. Deficient transport mechanism for the removal of acid monoamine metabolites from cerebrospinal fluid. *Brain Research*, 15, 522-524, 1969.
9. Bowers, M. B., Jr. Cerebrospinal fluid 5-hydroxyindoleacetic acid (5-HIAA) and homovanillic acid (HVA) following probenecid in unipolar depressives treated with amitriptyline. *Psychopharmacologia* (Berl.), 23, 26-33, 1972.
10. Brodie, H. K. H., Murphy, D. L., Goodwin, F. K., & Bunney, W. E., Jr. Catecholamines and mania: The effect of alpha-methyl-para-tyrosine on manic behavior and catecholamine metabolism. *Clinical Pharmacology and Therapy*, 12, 219-224, 1971.
11. Brodie, H. K. H., Sack, R., & Siever, L. Clinical studies of 5-hydroxytryptophan in depression. In: Barchas, J. and Usdin, E. (Eds.), *Serotonin and Behavior*. New York: Academic Press, 1973, pp. 549-559.
12. Butcher, L. L., & Engel, J. Behavioral and biochemical effects of L-dopa after peripheral decarboxylase inhibition. *Brain Research*, 15, 233-242, 1969.

13. Buus Lassen, J., Squires, R. F., Christensen, J. A., & Molander, L. Neurochemical and pharmacological studies on a new 5-HT-uptake inhibitor, F6 4963, with potential antidepressant properties. *Psychopharmacologia,* 42, 21-26, 1975.
14. Carlsson, A., Corrodi, H., Fuxe, K., & Hökfelt, T. Effect of antidepressant drugs on the depletion of intraneuronal brain 5-hydroxytryptamine stores caused by 4-methyl-α-ethyl-meta-tyramine. *European Journal of Pharmacology,* 5, 357-366, 1969. (a)
15. Carlsson, A., Corrodi, H., Fuxe, K., & Hökfelt, T. Effects of some antidepressant drugs on the depletion of intraneuronal brain catecholamine stores caused by 4, α-dimethyl-meta-tyramine. *European Journal of Pharmacology,* 5, 367-373, 1969. (b)
16. Carroll, B. J., Mowbray, R. M., & Davis, B. M. Sequential comparison of l-tryptophan with E.C.T. in severe depression. *Lancet,* 1, 967-969, 1970.
17. Coppen, A., Shaw, D. M., & Farrell, J. P. Potentiation of the antidepressive effects of a monoamine oxidase inhibitor by tryptophan. *Lancet,* 1, 79-81, 1963.
18. Coppen, A., Shaw, D. M., Herzberg, B., & Maggs, R. Tryptophan in treatment of depression. *Lancet,* 2. 1178-1180, 1967.
19. Coppen, A., Brooksbank, B. W. L., & Peet, M. Tryptophan concentration in the cerebrospinal fluid of depressive patients. *Lancet,* 1, 1393, 1972.
20. Deleon-Jones, F., Maas, J. W., & Dekirmenjian, H. Urinary catecholamine metabolites during behavioral changes in a patient with manic-depressive cycles. *Science,* 179, 300-302, 1973.
21. Deleon-Jones, F., Maas, J. W., Dekirmenjian, H., & Sanchez, J. Diagnostic subgroups of affective disorders and their urinary excretion of catecholamine metabolites. *American Journal of Psychiatry,* 132, 1141-1148, 1975.
22. Dunner, D. L. & Goodwin, F. K. Effect of l-tryptophan on brain serotonin metabolism in depressed patients. *Archives of General Psychiatry,* 26, 364-366, 1972.
23. Engelman, K., Lovenberg, W., & Sjoerdsma, A. Inhibition of serotonin synthesis by para-chlorophenylalanine in patients with the carcinoid syndrome. *New England Journal of Medicine,* 277, 1103-1108, 1967.
24. Fawcett, J., Maas, J. W., & Dekirmenjian, H. Depression and MHPG excretion: Response to dextroamphetamine and tricyclic antidepressants. *Archives of General Psychiatry,* 26, 246-251, 1972.
25. Feighner, J. P., Robbins, E., Guze, S. B., Woodruff, R. A., Jr., Winokur, G., & Munoz, R. Diagnostic criteria for use in psychiatric research. *Archives of General Psychiatry,* 26, 57-63, 1972.
26. Fieve, R. R., Platman, S. R., & Fliess, J. L. A clinical trial of methysergide and lithium in mania. *Psychopharmacologica,* 15, 425-429, 1969.
27. Fuller, R. W., Perry, K. W., & Molloy, B. B. Effect of an uptake inhibitor or serotonin metabolism in rat brain: Studies with 3- (p-trifluoromethylphenoxy)-N-methyl-3-phenylpropylamine (Lilly 110140). *Life Science,* 15, 1161-1171, 1974.
28. Fuller, R. W. & Molloy, B. B. Recent studies with 4-chloroamphetamine and some analogues. *Advances in Biochemical Psychopharmacology,* 19, 195-205, 1974.
29. Garelis, E., Young, S. N., Lal, S., & Sourkes, T. L. Monoamine metabolites in lumbar CSF: The question of their origin in relation to clinical studies. *Brain Research,* 79, 1-8, 1974.
30. Gershon, S., Hekimian, L. J., Floyd, A., Jr., & Hollister, L. E. α-Methyl-p-tyrosine (AMT) in schizophrenia. *Psychopharmacologia,* 11, 189-194, 1967.
31. Glassman, A. & Platman, S. R. Potentiation of a monoamine oxidase inhibitor by tryptophan. *Journal of Psychiatric Research,* 7, 83-88, 1969.

32. Goodwin, F. K., Brodie, H. K. H., Murphy, D. L., & Bunney, W. E., Jr. L-dopa, catecholamines and behavior: A clinical and biochemical study in depressed patients. *Biological Psychiatry*, 2, 341-366, 1970.

33. Goodwin, F. K., Post, R. M., Dunner, D. L., & Gordon, E. K. Cerebrospinal fluid amine metabolism in affective illness: The probenecid technique. *American Journal of Psychiatry*, 130, 73-79, 1973.

34. Goodwin, F. K. Discussion remark. In: Barchas, J. D., Hamburg, D. A. and Usdin, E. (Eds.), *Neuroregulators and Hypotheses of Psychiatric Disorders*. Oxford University Press (in press).

35. Gordon, E. K., Olivier, J., Goodwin, F. K., Chase, T. N., & Post, R. M. Effect of probenecid on free 3-methoxy-4-hydroxyphenylethylene glycol (MHPG) and its sulphate in human cerebrospinal fluid. *Neuropharmacology*, 12, 391-396, 1973.

36. Greenspan, K., Schildkraut, J. J., Gordon, E. K., Bar, L., Aronoff, M. S., & Durell, J. Catecholamine metabolism in affective disorders: III. 3-methoxy-4-hydroxyphenylglycol and other catecholamine metabolites in patients treated with lithium carbonate. *Journal of Psychiatric Research*, 7, 171-183, 1970.

37. Hamberger, B. & Tuck, J. R. Effect of tricyclic antidepressants on the uptake of noradrenaline and 5-hydroxytryptamine by rat brain slices incubated in buffer or human plasma. *European Journal of Clinical Pharmacology*, 5, 229-235, 1973.

38. Herrington, R. N., Bruce, A., Johnstone, E. C., & Lader, M. H. Comparative trial of l-tryptophan and E.C.T. in severe depressive illness. *Lancet*, 2, 731-734, 1974.

39. Jimerson, D. C., Gordon, E. K., Post, R. M., & Goodwin, F. K. Central noradrenergic function in man: Vanillylmandelic acid in CSF. *Brain Research*, 99, 434-439, 1975.

40. Karoum, F., Wyatt, R., & Costa, E. Estimation of the contribution of peripheral and central noradrenergic neurons to urinary 3-methoxy-4-hydroxyphenyl glycol in the rat. *Neuropharmacology*, 13, 302-312, 1975.

41. Korf, J., Praag, H. M. van, & Sebens, J. B. Effect of intravenously administered probenecid in humans on the levels of 5-hydroxy-indoleacetic acid, homovanillic acid and 3-methoxy-4-hydroxy-phenyl-glycol in cerebrospinal fluid. *Biochemical Pharmacology*, 20, 659-668, 1971.

42. Korf, J., Schutte, H. H., & Venema, K. A semi-automated fluorometric determination of 5-hydroxyindoles in the nanogram range. *Analyt. Biochem.*, 53, 146-153, 1973.

43. Levitt, M., Spector, S., Sjoerdsma, A., & Udenfriend, S. Elucidation of the rate-limiting step in norepinephrine biosynthesis in the perfused guinea pig heart. *Journal of Pharmacology and Experimental Therapy*, 148, 1-8, 1965.

44. Lidbrink, P., Jonsson, G., and Fuxe, K. The effect of imipramine like drugs and antihistamine drugs on uptake mechanisms in the central noradrenaline and 5-hydroxytryptamine neurons. *Neuropharmacology*, 10, 521-536, 1971.

45. Lloyd, K. J., Farley, I. J., Deck, J. H. N., & Hornykiewicz, O. Serotonin and 5-hydroxyindoleacetic acid in discrete areas of the brainstem of suicide victims and control patients. *Advances in Biochemical Psychopharmacology*, 11, 387-397, 1974.

46. Maas, J. W., Fawcett, J. A., & Dekirmenjian, H. Catecholamine metabolism, depressive illness, and drug response. *Archives of General Psychiatry*, 19, 129-134, 1968.

47. Maas, J. W., Fawcett, J. A., & Dekirmenjian, H. Catecholamine metabolism, de-

pressive illness, and drug response. *Archives of General Psychiatry,* 26, 252-262, 1972.

48. Maas, J. W. Biogenic amines and depression. Biochemical and pharmacological separation of two types of depression. *Archives of General Psychiatry,* 32, 1357-1361, 1975.

49. Matussek, N., Benkert, O., Schneider, K., Otten, H., & Pohlmeier, H. Wirkung eines Decarboxylasehemmers (Ro 4-4602) in Kombination mit L-dopa aut gehemmte Depressionen. *Arzneimittel-Fors.,* 20, 934-937, 1970.

50. Mendels, J., Frazer, A., Fitzgerald, R. G., Ramsey, T. A., & Stokes, J. W. Biogenic amine metabolites in cerebrospinal fluid of depressed and manic patients. *Science,* 175, 1380-1382, 1972.

51. Mendels, J., Stinnet, J. L., Burns, D., & Frazer, A. Amine precursors and depression. *Archives of General Psychiatry,* 32, 22-30, 1975.

52. Moses, S. G. & Robins, E. Regional distribution of norepinephrine and dopamine in brains of depressive suicides and alcoholic suicides. *Psychopharmacological Communications,* 1, 327-337, 1975.

53. Nagatsu, T., Hidaka, H., Kuzuya, H., & Takeya, K. Inhibition of dopamine-β-hydroxylase by fusaric acid (5-butylpicolinic acid) in vitro and in vivo. *Biochemical Pharmacology,* 19, 35-44, 1970.

54. Papeschi, R. & McClure, D. J. Homovanillic acid and 5-hydroxyindoleacetic acid in cerebrospinal fluid of depressed patients. *Archives of General Psychiatry,* 25, 354-358, 1971.

55. Pare, C. M. B., Yeung, D. P. H., Price, K., & Stacey, R. S. 5-Hydroxytryptamine in brainstem, hypothalamus and caudate nucleus of controls and of patients committing suicide by coal-gas poisoning. *Lancet,* 2, 133-135, 1969.

56. Post, R. M., Gordon, E. K., Goodwin, F. K., & Bunney, W. E., Jr. Central norepinephrine metabolism in affective illness: MHPG in the cerebrospinal fluid. *Science,* 179, 1002-1003, 1973.

57. Praag, H. M. van. A critical investigation of the significance of monoamineoxidase inhibition as a therapeutic principle in the treatment of depression. Thesis, Utrecht, 1962.

58. Praag, H. M. van & Leijnse, B. Die Bedeutung der Psychopharmakologie für die klinische Psychiatrie. Systematik als notwendiger Ausgangspunkt. *Nervenartzt,* 34, 530-537, 1964.

59. Praag, H. M. van & Leijnse, B. Neubewertung des Syndroms. Skizze einer funktionellen Pathologie. *Psychiat. Neurol. Neurochir.* (Amst.), 68, 50-66, 1965.

60. Praag, H. M. van, Uleman, A. M., & Spitz, J. C. The vital syndrome interview. A structured standard interview for the recognition and registration of the vital depressive symptom complex. *Psychiat. Neurol. Neurochir.* (Amst.), 68, 329-346, 1965.

61. Praag, H. M. van. The complementary aspects in the relation between biological and psychodynamic psychiatry. *Psychiatric Clinic,* 2, 307-318, 1969.

62. Praag, H. M. van & Korf, J. L-tryptophan in depression. *Lancet,* 2, 612, 1970.

63. Praag, H. M. van & Korf, J. Endogenous depressions with and without disturbances in the 5-hydroxytryptamine metabolism: A biochemical classification? *Psychopharmacologia,* 19, 148-152, 1971. (a)

64. Praag, H. M. van & Korf, J. Retarded depressions and the dopamine metabolism. *Psychopharmacologia,* 19, 199-203, 1971. (b)

65. Praag, H. M. van, Korf, J., Dols, L. C. W., & Schut, T. A pilot study of the predictive value of the probenecid test in application of 5-hydroxytryptophan as an antidepressant. *Psychopharmacologia,* 25, 14-21, 1972.

66. Praag, H. M. van, Korf, J., & Schut, T. Cerebral monoamines and depression. An investigation with the probenecid technique. *Archives of General Psychiatry,* 28, 827-831, 1973.
67. Praag, H. M. van & Korf, J. 4-Chloramphetamines. Chance and trend in the development of new antidepressants. *Journal of Clinical Pharmacology,* 13, 3-14, 1973.
68. Praag, H. M. van. Towards a biochemical typology of depression? *Pharmacopsychiatry,* 7, 281-292, 1974.
69. Praag, H. M. van, Burg, W. van den, Bos, E. R. H., & Dols, L. C. W. 5-Hydroxytryptophan in combination with clomipramine in "therapy-resistant" depression. *Psychopharmacologia,* 38, 267-269, 1974.
70. Praag, H. M. van & Korf, J. Central monoamine deficiency in depressions: Causative or secondary phenomenon. *Pharmakopsychiat.,* 8, 322-326, 1975.
71. Praag, H. M. van, Korf, J., Lakke, J. P. W. F., & Schut, T. Dopamine metabolism in depression, psychosis and Parkinson's disease or: The problem of the specificity of biological variables in behavior disorders. *Psychological Medicine,* 5, 138-146, 1975.
72. Praag, H. M. van & Korf, J. 4-Chloramphetamines. In: Usdin, E. & Forrest, I. S. (Eds.), *Psychotherapeutic Drugs.* New York: Marcel Dekker, Inc., 1976.
73. Praag, H. M. van. *Depression and Schizophrenia. A Contribution on Their Chemical Pathology.* New York: Spectrum Publications, 1976.
74. Praag, H. M. van. About the impossible concept of schizophrenia. *Comprehensive Psychiatry.* In press.
75. Praag, H. M. van. Indoleamines in depression. In: Barchas, J. D., Hamburg, D. A. & Usdin, E. (Eds.), *Neuroregulators and Hypotheses of Psychiatric Disorders.* Oxford University Press. In press.
76. Randrup, A. & Munkvad, I. Biochemical, anatomical and psychological investigation of stereotyped behavior induced by amphetamines. In: Costa, E. & Garattini, S. (Eds.), *Amphetamines and Related Compounds.* New York: Raven Press, 1970.
77. Redmond, E. E., Jr., Maas, J. W., Kling, A., Graham, C. W., & Dekirmenjian, H. Social behavior of monkeys selectively depleted of monoamines. *Science,* 174, 428-430, 1971.
78. Roos, B-E. & Sjöstrom, R. 5-Hydroxyindoleacetic acid and homovanillic acid levels in the cerebrospinal fluid after probenecid application in patients with manic-depressive psychosis. *Journal of Clinical Pharmacology,* 1, 153-155, 1969.
79. Ross, S. B. & Renyi, A. L. Inhibition of the uptake of tritiated 5-hydroxytryptamine in brain tissue. *European Journal of Pharmacology,* 7, 270-277, 1969.
80. Sack, R. L. & Goodwin, F. K. Inhibition of dopamine-β-hydroxylase in manic patients. *Archives of General Psychiatry,* 31, 649-654, 1974.
81. Sano, I. L-5-hydroxytryptophan (1-5-HTP)-therapie bei endogener Depression. *Münch. Med. Wschr.,* 144, 1713-1716, 1972.
82. Schildkraut, J. J. Norepinephrine metabolites as biochemical criteria for classifying depressive disorders and predicting responses to treatment: Preliminary findings. *American Journal of Psychiatry,* 130, 695-698, 1973.
83. Schildkraut, J. J., Keeler, B. A., Papousek, M., & Hartmann, E. MHPG excretion in depressive disorders: Relation to clinical subtypes and desynchronized sleep. *Science,* 181, 762-764, 1973.
84. Schildkraut, J. J. Biochemical criteria for classifying depressive disorders and predicting responses to pharmacotherapy: Preliminary findings from studies of norepinephrine metabolism. *Pharmacopsychiatry,* 7, 98-107, 1974.

85. Schildkraut, J. J. Depressions and biogenic amines. In: Hamburg, D. (Ed.), *American Handbook of Psychiatry*, VI. New York: Basic Books, 1975.
86. Schuckit, M., Robins, E., & Feighner, J. Tricyclic antidepressants and mono-amine oxidase inhibitors. *Archives of General Psychiatry*, 24, 509-514, 1971.
87. Schutte, H. H. Het metabolisme van serotonine in rattehersenen. Studies met radioactief gemerkt tryptofaan en toepassing van computersimulatie. Thesis, Groningen, 1976.
88. Shaw, D. M., Camps, F. E., & Eccleston, E. G. 5-Hydroxytryptamine in hindbrain of depressive suicides. *British Journal of Psychiatry*, 113, 1407-1411, 1967.
89. Shaw, D. M., O'Keeffe, R., MacSweeney, D. A., Brooksbank, B. W. L., Noguera, R. & Coppen, A. 3-Methoxy-4-hydroxyphenylglycol in depression. *Psychological Medicine*, 3, 333-336, 1973.
90. Shields, J. Genetic factors in neurosis. In: Praag, H. M. van (Ed.), *Research in Neurosis*. Amsterdam: Erven Bohn, B.V., 1976.
91. Shopsin, B., Wilk, S., Gershon, S., Davis, K., & Suhl, M. Cerebrosipnal fluid MHPG. An assessment of norepinephrine metabolism in affective disorders. *Archives of General Psychiatry*, 28, 230-233, 1973.
92. Shopsin, B., Wilk, S., Gershon, S., Roffman, M., & Goldstein, M. Collaborative psychopharmacologic studies exploring catecholamine metabolism in psychiatric disorders. In: Usdin, E. & Snyder, S. (Eds.), *Frontiers in Catecholamine Research*. New York: Pergamon Press, 1973, pp. 1173-1179.
93. Shopsin, B., Gershon, S., Goldstein, M., Friedman, E., & Wilk, S. Use of synthesis inhibitors in defining a role for biogenic amines during imipramine treatment in depressed patients. *Psychopharmacological Communications*, 1, 239-249, 1975.
94. Sjöström, R. & Roos, B-E. 5-Hydroxyindoleacetic acid and homovanillic acid in cerebrospinal fluid in manic-depressive psychosis. *European Journal of Clinical Pharmacology*, 4, 170-176, 1972.
95. Takahashi, S., Kondo, H., & Kato, N. Effect of l-5-hydroxytryptophan on brain monoamine metabolism and evaluation of its clinical effects in depressed patients. *Journal of Psychiatric Research*, 12, 177-187.
96. Trimble, M., Chadwick, D., Reynolds, E. H., & Marsden, C. D. L-5-hydroxytryptophan and mood. *Lancet*, 1, 583, 1975.
97. Tuck, J. R. & Punell, G. Uptake of (3H) 5-hydroxytryptamine and (3H) noradrenaline by slices of rat brain incubated in plasma from patients treated with chlorimipramine, or amitriptyline. *J. Pharm. Pharmacol.*, 25, 573-574, 1973.
98. Wålinder, J., Skott, A., Nagy, A., Carlsson, A., & Roos, B-E. Potentiation of antidepressant action of clomipramine by tryptophan. *Lancet*, 1, 984, 1975.
99. Westerink, B. H. C. & Korf, J. Determination of nanogram amounts of homovanillic acid in the central nervous system with a rapid semi-automated fluorometric method. *Biochemical Medicine*, 12, 106-115, 1975.
100. Wilk, S., Davis, K. L., & Thackes, S. B. Determination of 3-methoxy-4-hydroxyphenylcthylene glycol (MHPG) in cerebrospinal fluid. *Analytical Biochemistry*, 39, 498-504, 1971.
101. Wilk, S., Shopsin, B., Gershon, S., & Suhl, M. Cerebrospinal fluid levels of MHPG in affective disorders. *Nature*, 235, 440-441, 1972.
102. Wilk, S. Metabolism of biogenic amines in the central nervous system of man. Paper read at the Sixth International Congress of Pharmacology, Helsinski, 1975.

9

A Critical Overview of Diagnosis
in Psychiatry

ALVAN R. FEINSTEIN, M.D.

On a program that has produced so many stimulating but divergent viewpoints, I have the distinction of being not only the last speaker, but also the only one who has had no graduate exposure to psychiatric instruction and no formal experience in psychiatric practice. I can therefore make my remarks without inhibition, uncommitted to any particular school of thought and unencumbered by any intimate adventures in the clinical challenge of making psychiatric diagnoses.

The complex situation we have been contemplating can be greatly simplified if only we are allowed a bit of circular reasoning. At the root of the difficulty is the problem of deciding what is a diagnosis. We can dispose of that difficulty by defining a diagnosis as the name for a disease. We are now left with defining disease, which we can call a state of abnormal health. Abnormal health is readily defined as a departure from normal health. And then, completing the circle, normal health can be defined as the absence of disease.

I offer this circular oversimplification because it may be the only entity, of the many discussed at this symposium, on which an agreed consensus can be obtained. In the struggle to identify and name diseases, we are confronted with the facts that disease is an abstract concept, that it

The research presented in this paper was supported by PHS Grant Number 2-RO1-HS00408-07, from the National Center for Health Services Research and Development.

189

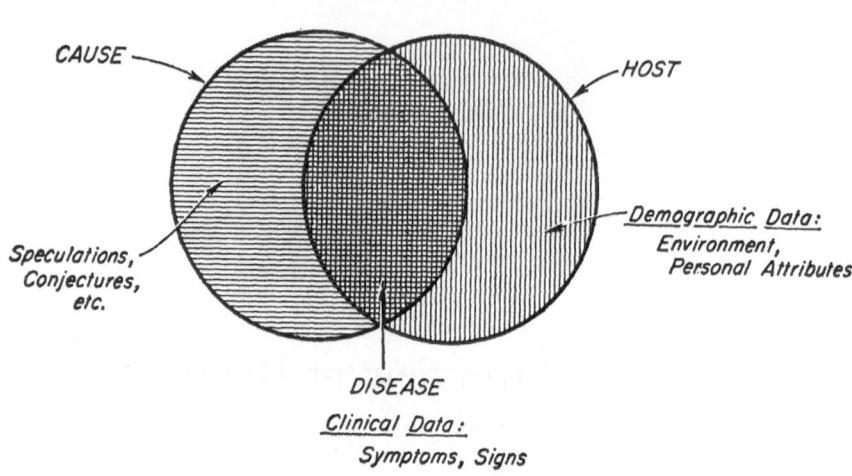

CAUSE

HOST

Speculations,
Conjectures,
etc.

Demographic Data:
Environment,
Personal Attributes

DISEASE

Clinical Data:

Symptoms, Signs

FIGURE 1. The nosologic model of disease in antiquity

remains abstract even if we re-title it with other names such as *ailment,
malady, sickness, illness, disorder,* or *derangement,* and that the only
workable definition of disease is that it represents whatever the doctors
of a particular era have defined a disease. For example, I know a way to
eliminate cancer overnight. How? In the same way that doctors eliminated
dropsy—by giving it another name. Dropsy is probably just as abundant
today as it was two centuries ago, but we now call it congestive heart
failure, or something else. Angina pectoris, which used to be a disease,
has been demoted in this century to being a symptom. The corresponding disease is now called coronary or ischemic heart disease.

EVOLUTION OF THE "MEDICAL MODEL"

If we go back to antiquity, the basic model of human ailments, as
shown in Figure 1, was that a cause of disease interacted with a human
host to form the particular set of discomforts, shown in the intersection
as a *dis-ease*—a clinically discomforted ease. The host was identified with
what might be called demographic data. The disease was observed directly
with what would today be called clinical symptoms and signs. But the
cause of disease was a subject of speculations and conjectures—beliefs
about deranged humors that could neither be demonstrated objectively

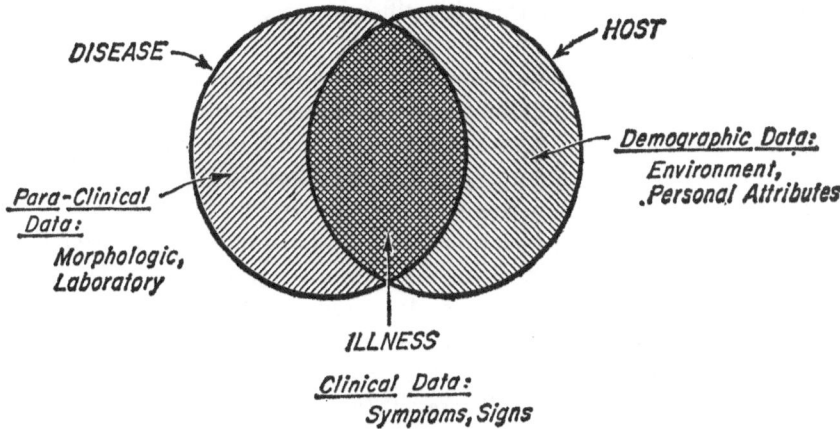

FIGURE 2. The current medical model of disease

nor proved experimentally. During the succeeding centuries, two major changes occurred in this model. The first, in the seventeenth century, was that Thomas Sydenham founded the discipline of nosology (1, 2) by insisting that diseases could be classified, that they often had constant predictable courses, and that certain individual manifestations, such as pain in the knee, pain in the big toe, and a tophus in the ear, were not separate diseases but could be clustered together as a single disease, gout. The second major change was the development of necropsy which provided morbid anatomic correlations for the clinically observed maladies, laboratory technology to provide chemical, physiologic and other objective evidence of the maladies, and animal experimentation to verify proposed pathways of etiology and pathogenesis.

As a result of these changes, the basic model was revised, as shown in Figure 2. What was earlier called a cause of disease became the disease itself, and its presence became identified with what might be called paraclinical data (2): information acquired away from the bedside (or couchside) by methods other than conventional clinical examination, and analyzed by the methods of radiography, pathology, and the phantasmagoria of modern laboratory tests. The host remained the same, still identified with demographic data. But the diverse symptoms, signs, and other clinical phenomena—which might be called the *illness*—were now left without a taxonomy for the formal identification needed for prognosis and therapy.

During these various changes, our ideas about disease and our names for disease have changed. The process of change was at its peak during the nineteenth century, and anyone who notes the hostile reception sometimes given today to proposals for alteration in psychiatric nomenclature can be assured that this is bland, compared to the acrimony and vilification with which physicians received the modifications offered in the nineteenth century. Dr. Grinker makes an eloquent plea (3) for the scientific necessity of preserving nosology and the idea of diagnosis itself. Less than a century ago he would have had to fight with the celebrated neurologist, Charcot, who said, "Il n'y a pas de maladies; il n'y a que des malades" (There are no diseases; there are only sick people).

Despite the opposition, the nosographic changers triumphed. We see the results in our current medical model of disease and in the nomenclature listed in the International Classification of Disease (ICD) that appears every ten years. In choosing to pursue this model and to cohabit intellectually with the taxonomic pundits who issue the ICD's decennial revisions, the nosographers of psychiatry may believe they will get some assured respectability, a certain amount of stability, or at least a good model. But the ICD, despite its widespread respectability, is neither stable nor a good model.

The decennial shifts in rubrics (4) have created havoc among attempts to perform scientifically credible comparisons of the occurrence of disease in different countries or different eras. In such chronic diseases as diabetes mellitus, arteriosclerosis, and cancer, the current ICD categories are prognostically worthless (2), and physicians concerned with estimating prognosis and evaluating therapy have had to create new mechanisms, such as staging systems, prognostic indexes, and other taxonomic tactics that help predict what a disease will do, rather than name what it is. On the few occasions where the actual usage of the ICD was specifically checked (4), the variability among the users was so great as to suggest that the domain of vital statistics was intellectually moribund.

Perhaps the greatest appeal of the so-called medical model for nosology is that the nomenclature is geared to pathogenesis and etiology. In general, whenever physicians succeeded in identifying what Claude Bernard called a *proximal* cause for a disease, we tried to change its name accordingly. And so the old clinical disease of *dyspnea* became the morbid anatomic disease, *pneumonia*. The morbid anatomic name became etiologically prefixed, when possible, resulting in terms such as *straphylococcal pneumonia*. Even in these cases, we haven't been consistent. When the old name serves the useful purpose of demarcating a spectrum, we preserve the old name. Thus, although the Group A steptococcus has been convincingly documented as an etiologic trigger for rheumatic fever, we still call the disease *rheumatic fever,* even though many patients with that malady are neither rheumatic nor febrile. Despite knowledge of the exact molecular structure that causes the disease, sickle cell anemia is still called *sickle cell anemia.*

The medical model of disease taxonomy may seem to have the appealing logic of etiology, but, in fact, the taxonomy is not logical at all. Its current array is an eclectically assembled, chronologic polyglot of different terms and ideas that reflect every layer of nosologic thinking and technologic data from antiquity to the present. Each layer has produced its own "new" diseases, while certain "old" diseases have persisted as veterans of nosographic nomenclature. Certain diseases are now named morphologically. They include the *infarctions, -omas, -lithiases, itises, -cytoses, -emias* and the many other rotund Latin phrases that our parents paid so much for us to learn in medical school. Other diseases are biochemical entities, such as *porphyria* and *hypogammaglobulinemia.* Yet others are abnormalities in physiology, such as *achalasia* and *atrial fibrillation.* Many names are those of microbial agents, such as *amebiasis* and *streptococcal infection.*

As examples of clusters, we have such disorders as *congestive heart failure* and the many syndromes of medicine, containing such eponyms as *Reiter's syndrome* and *Kleinfelter's syndrome.* Persisting old veterans of nomenclature are *rheumatic fever, gout,* and *coryza,* which is an ancient but eloquent name for the common cold. Some diseases are still named as physical signs. The patient says, "I've got a red rash with a lot of different shapes to it," and the doctor nods wisely and says, "Yes, you have *erythema multiforme*." Other diseases are named as symptoms. The patient says, "I've got an itchy rear end," and the doctor puts this into Latin as *pruritus ani.* Certain diseases, such as *chronic alcoholism* and *narcotic addiction,* are named according to habits. In the midst of all this illogical nomenclature, if psychiatrists seek solutions for their problems in nosology, the medical model offers respectability and tradition, but not necessarily a working, effective strategy.

TYPES OF CLASSIFICATION

To contemplate some of the basic issues in developing a workable strategy, we must first separate the two different intellectual activities that are involved in procedures of classification. The first is *taxonomic*. It consists of demarcating, defining, or otherwise establishing the categories that will be used for diagnosis. Thus, with an act of taxonomy, we decide that *chronic schizophrenia* is an acceptable name for a disease. The second procedure is *diagnostic*. It consists of providing rules of identification, enabling the selection of categories pertinent to a particular person. Taxonomy consists of providing definitions, but diagnosis requires operational identification.

For example, consider the entity called an adverse drug reaction. We can define it as the undesired effect of a drug given in appropriate dosage for an appropriate condition. This definition does not allow us, however, to make an operational identification or diagnosis of a drug reaction. For the latter decision, we need a set of criteria that will enable us to determine whether an observed episode of nausea or a skin rash should be attributed to a particular drug. The criteria would have to deal with the interpretation of such questions as whether the rash was part of the basic underlying disease, part of a superimposed disease, present before the candidate drug was used, or possibly associated with other drugs received concurrently, and whether the rash disappeared when the candidate drug was stopped or reappeared when the drug was resumed.

One of the most admirable features of the work done by Robert Spitzer's task force (5) in the preparation of DSM-III, whatever else one may think of it, is the attempt to provide criteria for operational identifications of diagnosis. The absence of such criteria is what has made the rest of the ICD such a shambles because it allowed the inconsistent variations with which the nomenclature is applied. Regardless of what happens to DSM-III, the production of operational identifications has been a pioneering, unique advance in nosology. Even if the taxonomy as a whole is disdained, the diagnostic operational criteria deserve attention, maintenance, suitable revision as needed, and, especially, gratitude and wild applause.

One can only hope that other workers in other branches of nosology will be equally enlightened and courageous in following the leadership of the psychiatric task force. In the field of diagnostic nosology, the establishment of operational criteria represents a breakthrough that is as obvious, necessary, fundamental, and important as the corresponding breakthrough in obstetrics and surgery when Semmelweiss, Oliver Wendell Holmes, and later on, Lord Lister, demanded that obstetricians and surgeons wash their hands before operating on the human body.

The more basic problems, however, are taxonomic rather than diagnostic. Before we decide on the algorithms, flow charts, or operational criteria that provide consistent diagnoses, we must choose the entities that will be sanctioned as categories of diagnosis. These issues in taxonomy will be the topic of the rest of my discussion.

In choosing an anchor or focus for the taxonomy, we can engage in two distinctly different types of nosologic reasoning. The first is to form names, designations or denominations for the observed evidence, and to confine ourselves exclusively to what has actually been observed. The second is to draw inferences from the observed evidence, arriving at inferential titles representing entities that have not actually been observed. For example, if a patient says "I have substantial chest pain, provoked by exertion, and relieved by rest," I, as an internist, perform a denomination if I designate this observed entity as *angina pectoris.* If I call it *coronary artery disease,* however, I perform an inference, since I have not actually observed coronary artery disease. If a radiologist looking at a coronary arteriogram or a pathologist cutting open the coronary vasculature uses the diagnosis *coronary artery disease,* the decision is a denomination. If the radiologist or pathologist decides that the coronary disease was caused by cigarette smoking or by a high fat diet, the etiologic diagnosis is an inference unless simultaneous evidence exists that the patient did indeed smoke or use a high fat diet. Even in this case, however, we have the *post hoc ergo propter hoc* problem of deciding whether and how causal inferences can be proved.

We can illustrate these issues, as shown in Figure 3, by noting that one form of classification consists of denominating the available evidence and confining the conclusion to that evidence. Or we can express the diagnostic conclusion in the form of an inference. The inference can occur by reasoning backward to an etiologic or pathogenetic cause preceding the ailment, or by a forward prediction, that estimates the prognosis or predicts the kind of treatment that will produce the best response.

For example, if a patient shows the manifest evidence of fever and coughing blood, my etiologic inference might be that the causal agent is

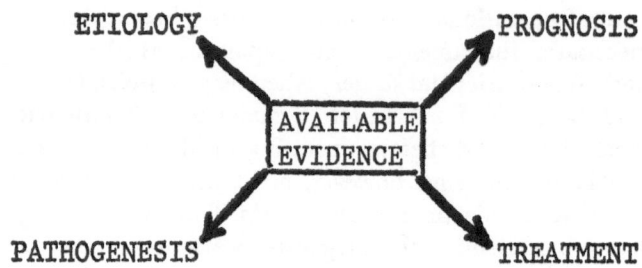

FIGURE 3. Patterns of Backward and Forward Inference
from Available Evidence

the tubercle bacillus. Pathogenetically, I may decide the blood came from
a cavity, produced in part, by inflammatory granulomas. Prognostically, I
might decide, according to this and other evidence, that the patient is
mildly or perhaps seriously ill. Therapeutically, I might decided that
this type of lesion responds well to streptomycin, and that bed rest or
isolation is or is not required for a good outcome.

The possible candidates for etiologic and pathogenetic mechanisms are
multiple and diverse. They include biologic aspects of microorganisms,
chemical reactions, anatomic configurations, and so on. They also include a series of physical agents, psychological sources, social factors, and a
large variety of familial, occupational, and other possible causes. As
prognostic indicators, we can choose to focus on survival, changes in
symptoms, changes in physical, social, or emotional function, costs, and
many other possibilities. In treatment, we can choose from many therapies, including pharmaceutical substances, surgery, radiation, the physician herself or himself, the patient, the family, and other people.

Regardless of whether a system of classification is denominational or
inferential, the system must be validated. Otherwise, it may be the
product of sheer speculation or arbitrary caprice. For example, when
Linnaeus classified animal organisms in the eighteenth century, his system of taxonomy was purely denominational. It was based mainly on
classifying animals according to observed mechanisms of locomotion and
reproduction. However, what gave the system a validity that makes it
endure was the later work of Charles Darwin in the nineteenth century.
It was Darwin, essentially, who gave the system an etiologic basis. He
pointed out that the phyla denominated by Linnaeus were produced by
an evolutionary process. Darwin's observations were later augmented by

embryologists who demonstrated that, for individual growth and development, ontogeny recapitulated phylogeny. Since the word validation means many things to many people, I shall explain that I use it here to denote whether a system of classification does what we want it to do, and how well it does it. What is the mechanism for concluding that a taxonomic system is good, effective, or appropriate?

METHODS OF VALIDATION

For an inference, the validation is external. We conclude something about a target that is outside the observed evidence, and we validate the conclusion by getting the direct evidence and seeing how it verifies or refutes the preceding conclusion. For example, if I conclude from a patient's history of angina pectoris, that he has coronary artery disease, my etiologic inference can be confirmed with suitable examination of other evidence by a radiologist or pathologist. And, if I predict he will be dead in three years, my prognostic estimation can be checked by noting the patient's state three years later.

In a denomination, the validation is internal, since we do not go outside our observed evidence. We can validate denominations by getting a consensual agreement from other professionals. We can try correlating the results of one system with the results of another, non-definitive system. (This is what happens when we check the results of a new anxiety scale against the results of some other established but non-validated scale for grading anxiety.) Finally, we can try to validate by purely mathematical techniques, seeing the way in which a particular scheme either reduces statistical variance and covariance, or optimizes some multivariate correlation or distance function.

The opportunity to perform an external validation is both the greatest strength and the greatest weakness of inferential classifications. The strength arises because we check against something that is outside our own intellectual machinations. This kind of external check provides the kind of fundamental scientific assurance that people seek in objective proof. The main weakness of the external validation is its requirement for something that is both external and acceptable to validate against. It is here that psychiatrists are so envious of the medical model of nosology and encounter so many problems in trying to develop their own. The easiest form of external validation is to use prognosis and therapy. Psychiatric patients, however, create a major difficulty in decisions about what kind of outcome is to be used as the main index of response. A classification system geared to survival alone may be substantially different from one geared to relief of symptoms or to general social function. To validate for etiology or pathogenesis is much more difficult than for prognosis and therapy, because it is necessary to provide not just evidence, but causal proof. If I say, as an outcome, that the patient is back at work, we have no quarrel in noting or accepting the evidence or the conclusion. If I say etiologically that his mother was nasty, you may accept my evidence of her nastiness, but you may demand better proof that her nastiness was the cause of his current psychic distress. In organic medicine, we have a double advantage in these matters. First, we have a vast array of paraclinical evidence (even in such simple things as X-rays) to document etiologic beliefs. Secondly, we have a large amount of animal experimental proof to support the etiologic beliefs. In psychiatry, we do not have very much objective paraclinical evidence, and our animal models are either nonexistent or too primitive to be of great value.

ETIOLOGIC DIFFICULTIES IN PSYCHIATRY

In search of etiology, psychiatrists are delighted and grateful when they can cite the organic part of an organic brain syndrome, but beyond the relatively small proportion of ailments that can receive these etiologic ascriptions, we are stuck. The various etiologic ideas provided by Freud and by other analytically oriented psychiatrists through psychodynamic theory have been perceptive, insightful, and often clinically useful. But none of the ideas has been accompanied by scientifically acceptable proof, and almost none of them is susceptible to tests by methods that would be clinically practical. As alternative sources of etiology and pathogenesis, psychiatrists have begun to do biochemical research, as described so well by van Praag (6), to investigate the leads offered by studies of monoamine metabolism and other metabolic substances. The search for hereditary, genetic factors has led to the interesting studies that were described by Wender (7) and Winokur (8).

These investigations of causal mechanisms are, of necessity, conducted under circumstances that require great perseverance and courage, and that would make most other scientists race back to the lab, to their hamsters and mice. The psychiatric etiologic investigators immediately encounter several major problems. First, they want to show the correlation of the biochemical or genetic results with the clinical maladies—but the clinical maladies may not be demarcated well enough to allow confidence in the quantified analyses. Secondly, when the items to be correlated consist of a psychiatric disease in a relative which has to be compared with psychiatric disease in a patient, the genetic relations may be badly blurred by the blurs in the diagnostic identifications. Finally, the kind of retrospective case-control study undertaken by Winokur and Wender is probably the only epidemiologic mechanism we can use to explore these relations. But the mechanism has many scientific imperfections, arising from problems of, perhaps unavoidable, bias both in the way the cases and controls are chosen and in their willingness to make themselves available for study (9).

The problem of etiologic proof for most psychiatric ailments is formidable. The magnitude of the difficulties suggests that if psychiatrists want an externally validated system of nosography, the anchor would have to be prognosis and therapy, rather than etiology and pathogenesis. This approach would be difficult to conduct. It would require the observation of patients for long periods of time and the collection of a great deal of follow-up data that have hitherto been neglected. The approach also might seem unscientific and contrary to the medical model. However, it currently offers the only hope of obtaining scientific proof for the inferences made with nosologic categories.

ACQUISITION AND INTERPRETATION OF EVIDENCE

In view of these difficulties in the quest for external validation, it is not surprising that so much of psychiatric diagnosis is denominational—a direct, noninferential classification of observed evidence. With this orientation, the questions become converted into issues of what evidence to collect, how to classify it, what to do with it and how to validate what has been done. Perhaps the most crucial source of evidence—even more important for psychiatry than for organic medicine—is the patient's history.

This information consists of the subjective statements that are volunteered by the patient spontaneously or in response to directive or nondirective forms of questioning. In view of the importance of this information, its acquisition must be reasonably standardized and reliable. We can therefore regard as a major scientific advance, the work described by Wing (10) in raising the quality and consistency of the information obtained by questionnaire interviews. This type of improvement in basic data can augment, not replace, the rest of the clinical interview, and can provide the kind of scientific confidence that is needed for credibility in the results of clinical or epidemiologic research.

As additional data, we have the so-called objective statements that come from observations by family and friends and also by physicians. One of the complaints sometimes lodged against psychoanalysis is that the exclusion of the family from the analytic interchange has served to exclude an important source of potentially valuable data. A distinctly objective set of manifestations consists of the physical signs that are available in posture, gestures, facial appearance, and vocal intonations, and, also, the limited amount of paraclinical evidence that is psychiatrically pertinent. Nevertheless, almost every psychiatrist with extensive experience is grateful for the biochemical test that allowed her or him, on at least one occasion, to scoop the internists who had failed to make the diagnosis of porphyria.

Finally, in a way that is, justifiably, almost unique in psychiatry, there is what might be called artifactual evidence. I use the word *artifact* here in its highest sense of human creativity, referring to entities that do not exist in nature. The music of Beethoven, the paintings of Picasso, and the architecture of Saarinen are all artifacts. In psychiatry, the artifactual evidence comes from special tests devised to provide a score for intangible attributes, such as intelligence and anxiety. Reitan (11) has given some superb examples of the kinds of procedures that he and his colleagues have invented for testing, scoring, and differentiating normal from abnormal brain function.

Once all this evidence has been acquired, we must decide what to do with it. We thus come to issues of interpretation. We can use designations, such as saying that a person who is pacing the floor is restless or anxious. We can decide about deviance by determining whether the findings are normal or abnormal. This is the type of decision that made Spitzer and his colleagues exclude normal grief from their array of psychiatric ailments. Having decided about deviance, we next determine pertinence. Which deviations are important? Which normal manifestations are important, even though not deviant? For example, it is abnormal to have one brown eye and one blue eye—but as long as vision is satisfactory, the deviation is unimportant. Conversely, many people with noses, breasts, or even genitals that are perfectly normal in appearance and in function have sought plastic surgery to alter the anatomy because of important psychic discontents. The decision about what is most importantly pertinent is nosologically crucial. It determines the information that will be preserved for subsequent analysis. In nosologic schemes from which a single diagnosis emerges, the decision about importance determines which among a series of candidate diagnoses will be selected.

The next three interpretations deal with attribution, combination, and consequences. In attribution, we make decisions about etiology and pathogenesis. In consequences, we predict what is going to happen, who will be affected, and what to do about it. The question of combination is intriguing: How do we form clusters or syndromes—particularly the ones that have no external inferential correlation? There now exist a series of statistical procedures for forming these clusters. The procedures go under such names as factor analysis, principal component analysis, cluster analysis, and a heroic computerized process called numerical taxonomy. The statistical procedures are all arbitrary; they all depend on mathematical principles that have no direct relationship to clinical reality. Further, they all have the major disadvantages, as noted by Wing (10), of being done without any clinical evaluations. Each of the different variables, from minor to major, is given the same weight. The combinational decisions are thus removed from the inconsistent comprehensibility of human judgments regarding importance and are relegated to the consistent inscrutability of mathematical caprices for correlation, variance, and distance.

A subdivision of the interpretive difficulties is the inconsistency with which decisions are made about concepts of deviance or deviation. One problem is that of impact. Who is affected by the deviation? The person alone, the family, or society? In psychiatry, we have many examples where the idea of deviance stems from society, not from individuals. The next problem relates to the way in which deviation is demarcated. Do we do it in a univariate statistical way, based solely on the person's location in an array of frequencies? This strategy, which is now being often used in the chemical laboratories of medical centers, can produce some odd results. We take a group of 1,000 healthy people and look at their frequency distribution curve for a chemical substance. We then use a statistical tactic to identify the inner 95% of the distribution as *normal* and the outer 5% as *abnormal*. Having chosen the 1,000 people originally because they were all normal, we then apply statistical strategies that will designate 50 of those people as abnormal!

To avoid such arbitrary peculiarities, we can reject the univariate statisticated concepts of deviation. We can insist on having a correlation, but we then must have something to correlate with. The correlation can be with the patient's current state of health, or even with a genetic state of health. For example, the sickle cell trait may not create any current or future difficulties for the health of its possessor, but its genes (if suitably mated) can create major problems for a member of a subsequent generation.

These are the kinds of difficulties we encounter at the elementary level of first order observation and characterization of data. At the next stage of reasoning, we take this characterized evidence and form the entities that become called diagnosis.

DIAGNOSTIC FORMULATIONS

Everything I have discussed so far has been concerned with taxonomy —with the creation of a set of available diagnostic categories. Let me now return to the usage of these categories—the work we do in identifying diagnoses for an individual patient. It is one thing to know that taxonomy provides categories that allow us to categorize eyes as *blue, brown,* or *other,* and hair as *black, brown, blonde,* or *other.* When we want to summarize the appearance of a particular person, however, do we mention eyes alone, or hair alone, or do we form a new combination, such as *fair complexion?*

This question brings us to issues in what might be called the depth and scope of diagnosis. By depth, I mean the amount of detail associated with a particular label. Do we label someone as *schizophrenia* alone, or *acute schizophrenia,* or *severe refractory acute schizophrenia?* By scope, I mean the number of different kinds of individual variables that are included in a diagnostic citation. For example, several of our speakers have pleaded for an enlarged scope of diagnostic citation, referring to multi-axial or multi-dimensional diagnoses. Wing (10) has suggested that the individual axes include one for acute symptoms, another for chronic impairments, and yet others for secondary handicaps and extrinsic disadvantages. Van Praag (6) wants separate axes for etiology, symptoms, prognosis, and pathogenesis. Stoller (12) has argued for inclusion of psychodynamics as either a separate axis or as a distinct component of pathogenesis. Spitzer (5) and his colleagues in DSM-III have, as of the moment, suggested five axes of classification: one for clinical psychiatric syndromes; a second for development or personality disorders; a third for nonmental disorders; a fourth for psychosocial stressors; and a fifth for level of adaptive functioning.

We are thus left with several different ways to do things, regardless of whether we do them by denomination or by inference. We can summarize a patient's diagnosis with a single "essence," depending on a hierarchy of ranked importance. This customary, traditional way of making diagnoses is the method advocated by Grinker (3) and it has the advantage, amidst its flaws, of being an evil we know and have borne, rather than an unfamiliar evil that may be even worse. A second procedure is to form clusters or syndromes, using either clinical or statistical judgments for the formations. The third procedure is an addition, not a supplement, to the other two. It contains multi-axial or multi-dimensional citations. All of these approaches are good and all of them are bad. We could argue interminably about the respective merits and demerits of each approach. We could also argue about the component entities that will be included or excluded as candidates when we select the things that will be essences, clusters, or members of the authorized elite of multi-axial categories.

Regardless of which side you take in the arguments, let me offer two sets of warnings about the rate of nosologic progress. Most medical students in North America look forward to learning about diagnosis by reading the Clinicopathologic Conferences that appear weekly in the *New England Journal of Medicine*. When those conferences were instituted in the 1920's by Richard Cabot (13), his main goal was nosologic. He thought American doctors were nosologically backward and he wanted them to begin using the new diagnostic terms that had been developing, mainly in Europe, for almost a century. Spitzer and his colleagues may have to institute some analogous conferences to arrange for the dissemination of DSM-III, and I hope he is prepared to wait a century to establish his immortality. As for multi-axial diagnoses, such a scheme was first proposed in 1922 by a criteria committee of the American Heart Association (14). There were five axes of classification: anatomy, etiology, physiology, functional state, and therapeutic recommendations. Thus, starting in 1928, doctors were no longer supposed to diagnose myocardial infarction. They were supposed to say something like: acute myocardial infarction; coronary thrombosis; normal sinus rhythm and cardiac compensation; unimpaired physical function; strict bed rest for next two days. I was taught to use that multi-axial system of classification when I was a medical student. Later I came East to work as a house officer at institutions where the multi-axial system had originated. By that time, 24 years later, the system had been apparently abandoned and the existing custodians of cardiac nomenclature were not using it. I would therefore urge Spitzer or any other nosologic innovators to be sure that the seeds are sown far away from home.

As the last speaker on this symposium, let me try to summarize what seem to be the six most prominent problems of psychiatric nosology.

1) The first is the absence of operational criteria and standardization for designating basic elements of observed "evidence," such as anxiety, tension, and hostility. All of the previously discussed operational criteria and other attempts at diagnostic standardization have been concerned with what is done after these basic elements have been designated, but there have been no attempts to bring consistency and uniformity to the basic designations themselves. Such terms as *anxiety, tension,* and *hostility* are really miniature diagnoses. In the absence of operational criteria, we have no idea of whether anxiety in Toronto means the same thing as anxiety in New York, and whether New York's anxiety is the same as New Haven's. Higher echelon diagnostic standards will remain scientifically unsatisfactory until the component basic elements have themselves been better standardized.

2) The second problem is the difficulty of external validation in the current absence of correlations either with etiologic evidence or with data for prognosis.

3) Third is the difficulty of validating "scales," "clusters," and other formulations of data. In the absence of documented etiologic or prognostic evidence and in the absence of standard diagnoses, the kinds of tests created by Reitan and the questionnaire evidence assembled by Wing do not have equally good information to relate to.

4) Fourth is the difficulty in establishing meaning or value for etiologic or pathogenetic research in absence of diagnostic or prognostic correlation.

5) Without external correlations and validations, the fifth problem is that of denominational diagnoses. They may be the product of unstandardized caprices for clinical choices of an "essence," or they may emerge from arbitrary mathematical rituals used to demarcate "factors" or "clusters."

6) Finally, although we all recognize the crucial need for multiple axes of classification, we encounter major disagreements about which axes to preserve and unresolved uncertainties about which data to include.

Amid these handicaps, which currently seem almost insurmountable, the innovative or controversial proposals of DSM-III become somewhat like the famous Russian dancing bear. Of course, the bear does not dance well, but the remarkable thing is that the bear dances at all. It is easy to be adversely critical about any approach to nosology, just as one can comment critically on what we have observed in this symposium: the disparate beliefs, the adverse approaches, the scientific discrepancies, and even the illegible lantern slides. Nevertheless, the most striking and constructive thing about this symposium is its very occurrence. It indicates that psychiatrists have begun quite seriously to recognize and to approach the massive problems of nosography. Of course, you do not yet have solutions, but you have begun to acknowledge their absence and you have begun to identify the problems that must be solved. I admire and congratulate you for having done so. The nosographic problems are almost as great in the world of so-called organic disease, but we nonpsychiatrists persistently evade them and complacently ignore them.

The medical model of diagnosis to which you may aspire is in almost as great a need of improvement as the existing psychiatric catalog, but we continue to escape the clinical challenges that confront us. The escapes usually take the form of hoping that some other investigator, working in some other domain, will take care of everything. We may thus fervently believe that the biochemist has the answers, and if not, the biophysicist may have them. This belief requires the additional faith that afterward, we will find questions to go with the answers. A different avenue of escape is to believe that the computer has the answers, and if not, the statistician may have them. For this type of escape, we have faith that afterward, we will find something to do with the data. If all these fail, there is the greatest escape of all—the hope that maybe the pharmacologist will find something that will work.

My last set of comments is provoked by two qualifications: my presence here as an alleged expert in nosology and my status of being unfettered by an intimate knowledge of psychiatric practice. I shall take advantage of both these qualifications to make some suggestions about the most effective ways you might proceed in trying to improve psychiatric nosography.

I would urge that you concentrate on raw evidence and on standardization of elements of evidence. In gearing your nosography to an inferential anchor, you might concentrate on verifiable inference, such as response to treatment, but particularly on natural prognosis and clinical course, which can be established without regard to changes in therapeutic technology. You might also concentrate on correlating observed evidence with target inferences or with other clearly stipulated targets. You should avoid arbitrary demarcations, simplification for the sake of simplifying, and the kinds of traditional clinical escapes that I mentioned earlier. Be sure to heed the Queen's advice to Alice in Wonderland: Consider everything. And finally, as you struggle with the magnitude and complexity of this enormous challenge, don't get too depressed.

REFERENCES

1. Faber, K. *Nosography in Modern Internal Medicine.* New York: Paul B. Hoeber, Inc., 1923, p. 74.
2. Feinstein, A. R. *Clinical Judgment.* Huntington, New York: Robert E. Krieger Co., Inc., 1974.
3. Grinker, R. R., Sr., this volume, 69-83.
4. Feinstein, A. R. Clinical epidemiology: II. The identification rates of disease. *Annals of Internal Medicine,* 69, 1037-1061, Nov., 1968.
5. Spitzer, R. L., Sheehy, M., & Endicott, J., this volume, 1-24.
6. Van Praag, H. M., this volume, 153-189.
7. Wender, P. H., this volume, 109-127.
8. Winokur, G., this volume, 128-152.
9. Feinstein, A. R. Clinical Biostatistics: XX. The epidemiologic trohoc, the ablative risk ratio, and "retrospective" research. *Clinical Pharmacology and Therapy,* 14, 291-307 (March-April), 1973.
10. Wing, J. K., this volume, 84-108.
11. Reitan, R. M., this volume, 42-68.
12. Stoller, R. J., this volume, 25-41.
13. Cabot, R. L. Quoted in W. A. Hunter: A study of diagnostic errors in clinico-pathologic conferences at the Massachusetts General Hospital during a 25-year period. *Permanente Foundation Medical Bulletin,* 10, 306, 1952.
14. New York Association. *Criteria for the Classification and Diagnosis of Heart Disease.* 1st Edition. Boston: Little, Brown & Company, 1928.

Panel Discussion

Following the presentation of the papers, the participants in the symposium met for a panel discussion during which they discussed issues that had come up during the meeting. In addition they responded to questions from the audience.

THE CONCEPT OF DIAGNOSIS OR DISORDER

Spitzer: Although Dr. Stoller* and I had several discussions a few hours prior to his talk there was a misunderstanding which came out in his paper. And I would just like to clear it up since it relates to an issue that has caused a lot of concern. This has to do with the requirement of distress in making a diagnosis of one of the sexual deviations which we now call the sexual arousal disorders. Dr. Stoller said that the position of the DSM-III task force was that those conditions required distress before they could be considered diagnostic entities. What he was recording was a decision the task force had made 14 months ago and quickly abandoned. Since then we have been spending all our efforts trying to convince people that we really have abandoned that position. There was one category—homosexuality—which, as you know, has been the subject of a lot of controversy; that category is not considered a diagnosis unless it is accompanied by distress. Within the last two weeks we have coined the term *homodysphilia* which refers to homosexuals who are distressed by their homosexual arousal. With the exception of

---

* Dr. Stoller's paper published in this volume takes this discussion into account.

that category, the other sexual deviations or sexual arousal disorders as we call them are considered diagnostic entities regardless of whether or not they are accompanied by the complaint of distress.

Stoller: I am only asking Dr. Spitzer to consider whether he wouldn't put heterosexuality in there also.

Spitzer: Actually we do have a wastebasket category which we've called psychosexual distress disorder, not elsewhere classified. We list eight examples in the latest draft of DSM-III, including women who wish they were homosexual and not heterosexual and you can think of other categories of such ill-defined conditions.

Regarding another comment of Dr. Stoller's: I think it is useful to distinguish different levels of comprehension in terms of a diagnostic entity or the term disorder that we used. We have suggested that the term disease be reserved for those disorders where we have a specific aetiology or pathophysiological process. In that sense, obviously, we don't have many diseases in psychiatry. When Dr. Stoller says that if we don't understand aetiology, we don't really have a true diagnosis, he ignores the fact that in diagnosis we are talking about varying degrees of validity. Although we don't have many fully validated diagnostic entities, I don't think we should assume that we are not dealing with legitimate diagnostic entities when we don't know the aetiology or the pathophysiological process. Manic depressive illness is certainly an example of a diagnostic entity where we do not know the aetiology and/or the pathophysiology, but it is a distinct clinical condition. We have a rather specific treatment for it. In that sense it is not unlike other areas of medicine where we frequently have a diagnostic entity that we can treat without having a complete understanding of aetiology. I guess it's partly a question of presentation and tone. Maybe I am overly sensitive to the anti-psychiatric or the anti-psychiatry movement which is always attempting to cut us off from the rest of medicine, and perhaps I am being somewhat defensive. With anything that sounds as if it might be used to suggest that we are fundamentally different from the rest of medicine, I feel called upon to respond to it.

SPECTRUM AND BORDERLINE CONCEPT

Grinker: I don't think it will be any surprise to you that I disagree with my colleagues Drs. Winokur and Wender. As I said in my presentation, spectrum defines certain illnesses within the family structure which are predisposing to the index illness that is being studied. For example, Dr. Winokur talks about two markers, alcoholism and asocial personality, and he is very clear that these are not the disease that he is studying. Now before I would accept the fact that these markers are really significant within the families of manic depressives, and in some way concerned with the development of the disease in the index subject, I would have to accept more than his statement, "We made a rigorous definition." Now I don't know what a rigorous definition of alcoholism is and I don't know anybody who has made one. Nor do I know what a rigorous definition of asocial personality is, since it varies in universities and in teaching centers in different parts of the country. Furthermore, he says that a patient with anxiety is excluded. Now clinical experience shows that frequently anxiety is present as the patient is going into a depression and also appears as the patient is coming out of a depression. Anxiety and depression are closely linked.

I also have objections to Dr. Wender's representation of the spectrum concept in schizophrenic studies. In the first place, he and his colleagues have utilized chronic schizophrenia. He does not accept the diagnosis of acute schizophrenia, rather. calling it reactive schizophrenia, which wipes it out of any genetic proposition. We know if you follow acute schizophrenic patients over long periods of time, as Manfred Bleuler has done, that attack after attack is associated with a decrease in competence and social abilities, and an increase in thought disorder. These patients frequently become chronic. What Dr. Wender has done is to utilize what is called pseudo-neurotic schizophrenia (which is a bad name to begin with) as one of the members of the spectrum rather than as a schizophrenia itself. In the follow-up study of the patients called pseudo-neurotic schizophrenics by Hoch and Polatin, about 40% of them ended up in state hospitals, indicating that for the most part they were schizophrenic.

Wender also uses the term borderline schizophrenia. In my view you can't be borderline schizophrenic. You can be borderline psychotic; but psychotic doesn't mean schizophrenia. There are many other kinds of psychoses. Dr. Wender defines so-called borderline schizophrenia utilizing what really has been the language of Kalmann. If you do that, then you are more likely to be talking about schizophrenia. However, looking at the literature from the beginning, the term borderline was applied to those psychiatric entities for which I have decided to use the language of Robert Knight et al. Throughout the literature, borderline refers to an individual who has certain specific characteristics and does not display the thought disorder or the psychotic breaks found in schizophrenia. If the definition of the borderline is not that of schizophrenia and is still used for one of the members of the spectrum, I would like to remind Dr. Wender that studies of the families of borderline patients show characteristics very similar to the borderline. They are not schizophrenic, and the descendants of a particular borderline very frequently have the same kind of personality and character disorder as that person.

I think you have to be very clear that there are two divisions when you tackle any syndrome. One is the core process, as in the processes that characterize schizophrenia. We know, for example, that hallucinations do not characterize schizophrenia. They are not essential to the diagnosis of schizophrenia, although they may be present. Similarly, if you characterize the core process of the borderline as horrible loneliness and the absence of the ability to receive any kind of emotional sustenance from another human being, then one can recognize that drug addiction and alcoholism represent secondary symptoms which are not an expression of the borderline condition, but represent an attempt to defend against the core process. So on two grounds I object to the spectrum concept: first, the use of the chronic to the exclusion of the acute; and second, the misuse of the term borderline schizophrenia.

Questions from the Audience

Please give the clinical features of borderline schizophrenia.

How do you relate your conception of borderline schizophrenia to Roth et al.'s recently published suggestions that the spectrum should be narrow?

Is the schizophrenia spectrum indeed specifically linked to schizophrenia or is it more generally a label for psychological vulnerability? In addition, do such people have more phsyical illness and do they degenerate more rapidly? Is this possibly a manifestation of "poor protoplasma"?

Wender: The fact that the word "spectrum" makes Dr. Grinker uncomfortable is irrelevant to its usefulness. When I discussed the acute or schizophrenic form of psychoses, my colleagues and I were fully aware of Langfeld's 1938 study which indicated that one-third of these people go on to develop chronic schizophrenia. I was really indicating the fact that in Scandinavia and Europe in general, most people tend to regard the pure form of the disorder as either psychogenic or reactive. Now one of the major points I tried to make is that borderline is an adjective and without having it modify a noun one does not know what one is talking about. Borderline might mean borderline schizophrenia, borderline affective disorder, borderline sociopathy, borderline alcoholism. Since the word originally was used in reference to schizophrenia-like individuals, I thought it useful to fully extrapolate the term and provide the noun as well as the adjective. With regard to Dr. Grinker's assertion about Hoch and Polatin's follow-up, not *40%* but *10%* of their subjects wound up in the mental hospital some time in their life. Now one of the other points I tried to make very clearly and explicitly was that we had begun with Hoch and Polatin's criteria. What we found is that human beings are exceedingly variable, and that there were very few individuals who met all these criteria, but many people who approximated them. Using my analogy of wines: There were Beaujolais and there were burgundies and there were a variety of other red wines which had more or less similar tastes. But the proof of the diagnostic pudding was the fact that (a) we had high inter-rater reliability and (b) that we found that the usefulness of the concept was validated by the fact that this syndrome was found to be increased only among the relatives of schizophrenic patients. We then collaborated with Dr. Spitzer and others to get an operational definition, and I believe he will address himself to this point.

I think it is important to indicate that in the first study I mentioned —the one in which we investigated the biological relatives of adopted schizophrenics—the only disorders we found increased in frequency were in the schizophrenic spectrum as compared to the biological relatives of the controls. We did not find increased affective disorder nor did we find increased sociopathy. The other point I have to mention in relation to Dr. Grinker's study is that this was a logical bootstrap operation. We generated the concept as well as validating it, because we were starting with the relatives of schizophrenic patients. But one need not call them borderline schizophrenics; one can simply describe their characteristics. In Dr. Grinker's study the patients entered the sample in a very different way, which would accept anybody who is a little crazy but not too crazy, and who therefore might not bear any relationship whatsoever to schizophrenia. We have currently completed an adoptive study of the relatives of individuals with a variety of forms of affective disorder and we have not yet analyzed the data. It is my expectation that we will probably not find an increase of either sociopathic or affective disorder among the biological relatives of these adopted depressive subjects. The indication to me so far is that these diseases or disease groupings move rather cleanly and together. Dr. Spitzer, would you like to comment on your and Jean Endicott's recent work?

Spitzer: This is a test of my long-term memory, but I have tried to jot down the six items that we found after reviewing the cases and comparing them with the control cases. We developed a series of items, then we saw which items actually discriminate the groups. We found that we could identify, I believe, six items and that virtually all of the cases considered borderline by Wender, Kety, and Rosenthal had at least three of these six items. The first item was undue social anxiety or social sensitivity or social isolation; second was ideas of reference or paranoid ideation; third was signs of what we referred to as mild thought disorder—that is, it would not be full thought disorder, but there were signs of cognitive slippage of one kind or another; fourth was affective impoverishment during the interview; fifth was unusual perceptual experiences; and the sixth was signs of magical thinking short of delusional ideation. I think it is interesting that almost all of those signs are really mild forms of characteristic schizophrenia symptomatology.

van Praag: I think all the American discussions using the term borderline psychosis can be related to the term psychogenic psychosis, as it is called in Europe. As far as I remember, it is not a symptomatological concept. The term psychogenic psychosis in Europe is based on, let's say, three findings: first of all, the presence of sociogenic and psychogenic factors; secondly, the presence of a more or less clear-cut neurotic premorbid personality; and finally, accessibility to psychotherapy. So I believe all authors in Europe agree that there is a considerable overlap in symptomatology, but I think the concept was introduced not on symptomatological criteria but on premorbid personality and psychogenic factors.

Grinker: I would like to answer with just four brief sentences. The question of borderline—to what? It is quite true we don't say to what, but we use the term borderline because it's in the literature. Once you get something like that in the literature, you can't change it. Second sentence: The term borderline was used first to designate something not quite insane; it had nothing to do with schizophrenia. Third sentence is that the six characteristics mentioned by Dr. Spitzer are not the characteristics of a borderline; if you want to use those characteristics, then you have another entity called borderline schizophrenia (but I object to the use of the term borderline in that respect). And the next sentence with which I will close is that I don't think we can talk about either a totally genetic condition or totally reactive; I think they are both equally biogenetic and psychologically reactive.

Wender: I would just like to make one answer to that and let Dr. Winokur pick up on the rest. It is interesting that in our four studies of adopted schizophrenics we have not found one datum indicating psychological etiological components. It is always good to say that things are multi-determined, but so far we have not been able to find any evidence of psychological factors playing a role in the genesis of the schizophrenias.

Winokur: I want to thank Dr. Grinker for having raised some questions that give me an opportunity to expand on what I mean by rigorous definition. Every patient in the last parts of the studies met the Feighner criteria for alcoholism, antisocial personality and depression. Now your next question should be, "Are they reliable?" The answer is they were reliable in a series of reliability studies at Washington University and in the progeny of the Feighner criteria, namely the Research Diagnostic Criteria of Spitzer et al. Are they valid diagnoses? I think they are valid diagnoses because using the Feighner criteria there are a series of adoption studies showing a genetic factor in alcoholism, antisocial personality. The study of alcoholism was done by Goodwin, Guze, Hermansen, Schulsinger and myself. The study of antisocial personality (not *a*social personality, by the way) was done by Raymond Crowe and the study of depression was done by Remi Cadoret. And in all these, using these particular sets of reliable criteria, you also find that there is a genetic factor using adoption study methodology. That is what I meant by rigorous definition of the illnesses. Does that prove that the spectrum disease exists? No! There is only one way to prove it exists and that is by the finding of a specific marker, such as a specific biological marker like α-haptoglobin or C3 or group of specific components or ABO or RH. We have some material that indicates that is true and I presented that material to you. Actually we have some more material which I didn't present which proves the spectrum exists. In our definition of the spectrum, a number of clinical syndromes are given equal weight. Alcoholism is equal to depression which is equal to antisocial personality and it is simply a difference in the way it manifests itself within different sexes.

Next, Dr. Grinker brought up an interesting point relating to the methodology. He said, why did you throw out anxiety, because lots of times anxiety may predate the making of another diagnosis? The answer to that is simple. We had a group of patients who fitted the depression spectrum. We had another group of subjects who were considered normal. We then took the normal group and compared it with the group considered to be spectrum cases, and we ran the X^2 box with the said pairs with the specific markers, and it showed a positive finding. We then added the anxiety neurotics and the hysterics and the various other diagnoses that appeared on both sides and it turned out they looked like the normals. So they are not part of the schizophrenia part of the depression spectrum. They are part of normality as far as this particular study is concerned. By normality we mean they are not simply part of the depression spectrum. That's why they belong with the normals. They are not normal in terms of diagnosis, but they are also not part of the depression spectrum.

Feinstein: I am very troubled by the concept of the borderline schizophrenic. I am very confused by the word borderline. Is it sort of like saying borderline pregnancy, is it borderline survival, or is it being used to mean a very mild state? If it means a very mild state, why not use the word mild? But the word borderline I find very confusing and it seems to me, as an external observer of the nomenclature, that that is a very weak spot. I am troubled by some of the comments on the genetics. In the other kinds of genetic studies, the disease entity is clearly demarcated and there is essentially no question about what it is. It's cancer or it's sickle cell anemia and there is general agreement as to what the disease marker is. And then you go track down that marker in the families. In that circumstance you might find some people who have the trait but not the full-blown clinical manifestations, because you do in fact have agreement on the marker and you can identify it. Given the extraordinary difficulties that you have here with identifying the disease itself and given the absence of a marker, what is it that enables you to have such total confidence in these numbers, in the precision with which you can say 34 out of 239? I admire that precision enormously, but I have grave doubts about what confidence one can give to the particular intellectual state that lies behind the numbers.

Spitzer: Regarding the term "borderline," the reason it has stuck around is that it seems to serve a function. I think the function that it serves is that if we were to use the alternative form "mild," it would indicate something we are not prepared to say—that these things that we have called borderline are mild forms of the disorder schizophrenia. Now I think that Wender, Kety, Rosenthal believe they really are mild forms, but many of us can only note that there are some similarities between those characteristics and symptoms that precede the onset of schizophrenia or are residual symptoms. So we see individuals who have some of these characteristics. They never seem to have the full-blown (or they rarely develop the full-blown) condition which it resembles. It is a relatively stable condition. So it is as if someone was going across the border but decided not to move. And I think that's our dilemma, and until we know more, I don't know that we are going to find a better term. That's why I've resigned myself to having the term borderline personality disorder in DSM-III, because I can't think of a better term.

Winokur: And I, Dr. Spitzer, am very unhappy about it because we have shown that some characteristics move in common while we don't know if the other 6 to 12 out of 18 characteristics that have been covered do or not. I would suggest that we call the Rosenthal, Wender, Kety syndrome "Hassenpfeffer's syndrome" which will have no meaning to any one else.

Spitzer: Well I would be glad to do that if we have any evidence that "Hassenpfeffer's syndrome" was discrete from the other borderline items. I don't think your study provides us with that data because I don't think your interviewer was looking for those other items.

Wender: That's hard to say because our interviewer was also aware of the general, broad, fuzzy types of problems that have been called borderline in the past.

Spitzer: But your interviewer had certain categories of information he was always looking for. He was always talking about whether or not there were signs of magical thinking, thought disorder, and impoverishment of affect.

Grinker: He wasn't looking for affective variations that influence impulsivity or a whole variety of other characteristics, which have been asserted by some to be related to borderline. Everyone knows you just simply cannot change these diagnostic terms easily. Now, in our experience there are four separate subgroups of the borderline state. They don't progress, and their characteristics remain constant; they don't move one group to another. One group has been called "psychotic character" because, occasionally, in the midst of tremendous anger their ego functions dissolve and they become psychotic for a few hours or a few days, but recover quickly. The second is what we call "the core of the borderline": They attempt to make positive relations with other people, get angry, leave the scene, become lonely and despondent, and attempt to return. The third group is the one that Helene Deutsch described 25 years ago as *"as-if"* characters. And the fourth group is more like the neurotic and the clinical depression where the individual seeks out a maternal figure but can't stand her when she gets it. Then she moves away. They are mostly women. I don't think we are going to solve this problem of the borderline at this meeting. And I don't think the Washington University establishment is going to accept that. The second thing I would like to say is that sometimes I feel at a meeting like this that I am in a never-never land. For example, Dr. Winokur has stated there is no psychological basis at all and Dr. Wender said there are no psychological factors in the aetiology of the schizophrenias. Now can anybody believe that?

Wender: I'll have to interrupt you because I am being misquoted and it may mislead the audience. I said our studies have failed to show this using our data.

Winokur: I said I believe we can't prove it.

Grinker: Alright. You're both hedging! And I say to you that, given a specific biogenetic make-up, the majority of precipitating factors are psychological. If you want to dispute that, show me the evidence.

GENETIC LINKAGE

Spitzer: This is a question for Dr. Winokur, but I would hope Dr. Feinstein might also comment. It seems to me that the logic you have been proposing is, that if one can demonstrate that two forms of a condition have different genetic components, then one has demonstrated two disease entities. I would question whether that logic really makes sense. Could not one also say that one is showing that there are different host factors which affect the likelihood of a single disease entity being expressed? For example, couldn't one explain your data by a host factor which determines whether or not you are likely to get the single illness depression at an earlier age and perhaps that host factor also makes you more vulnerable to alcoholism and antisocial personality? What I am really concerned with is, how we know when we have a distinct disease entity? And are you not ignoring host factors in your conceptualization of a disease entity?

Winokur: Well I can answer that, I think. It's something I have done a lot of thinking about. The fact is that both groups that manifest themselves as depression spectrum and a pure depression look alike. Both of them fill the Feighner criteria. Both of them will no doubt fill the Research Diagnostic Criteria too. So, in that sense they are the same illness. Then we find that there is a different family background. And now we find that there is a likelihood that there is a different genetic factor. The only way you could consider them the same illness would be if the entire concept of the illness was polygenic. And you would have to say the depression spectrum needed more genes than the pure depressive and was therefore a more severe disease, starting earlier and affecting more family members. That would be a way of explaining it. But the fact is I don't think you can do that as long as you find an individual genetic marker is manifesting itself in linkage with only one of them. It shows a real specificity. Now I suppose, rather than argue the point of whether they are one or two diseases, maybe the logical conclusion is there is gentic heterogeneity. I suppose nobody will argue with that. Now that could be true whether there were more genes or fewer genes; but in fact the α-haptoglobin and C3 are only associated with depression spectrum disease. When you do a similar kind of study with the pure depressive group, they are not linked. Therefore, there is certainly genetic heterogeneity. To me that's disease heterogeneity. More than one disease. I admit that they look alike clinically.

Berg (Questioner from the audience): Dr. Winokur, the point that I want to raise with you relates to the question of sex linkage in certain groups of the affective disorders. I think that one ought to find more precisely what type of sex linkage one is talking about. You are obviously not referring to a gene linked to the Y chromosome; you are obviously not referring to a gene lined to the X chromosome, and you are not talking of an X-linked recessive disability such as hemophilia. What you suggest is a factor relevant in the causation at least of some types of the affective disorders in the context of X-linked dominance. One of the puzzles that I have in regard to X-linked dominance is that patterns of transmission ought to be so precise that the evidence in favor of an X-linked dominant circumstance would be more overwhelming than your data suggest. For instance, you quite rightly point out that if an affected father married a normal mate, none of the sons of that union could be affected. By the same token, if one was dealing with an X-linked dominant and an affected father had children by a normal mother, you would expect every daughter to be affected. Unless such facts emerge from the pedigree studies, I think it would be extremely difficult to argue very vigorously in favour of an X-linked dominant proposition.

The other problem is that if one investigates patterns of transmission of genetic disabilities in terms of deviance, one simply doesn't find clearcut evidence of X-linked dominance. There are several approximations to that state of affairs, where there are so-called intermediate genes with manifestations both in males and females, but not identical manifestations. As far as I know, there isn't a single instance where there is a clearcut picture of X-linked dominant inheritance involving a single dominant gene. My real question is whether you would agree that if one was dealing with an X-linked dominant gene, the evidence in favor of such transmission would be more overwhelming in terms of a pedigree data than in fact it is.

Winokur: I used the term X-linkage rather than sex linkage all the way through, which indicated that it was X-link, not Y. Now there is only one Y-link possibility that I can find and that is hairy ears, or something of that sort, and I don't think we need worry about that too much. As Dr. Berg asks, "Why is it not more dramatic? An ill father should have all ill daughters and he should have no ill sons." Well, my calculation from the epidemiological data indicates that only 51% of families are X-linked. Therefore, if you take a group of manic patients into a family study, you are going to have a vast mixture and nothing is going to be striking about it. The thing I think fortunate was that in our original study we must have "lucked" into that kind of group—namely, that they were mostly X-linked, and the other ones were not informative so it didn't wash out. Now why don't all the daughters become ill? I don't know. My guess is that not everybody shows the pathophysiology associated with the genes. That's called lack of penetrance. As far as I am concerned, it's a useless word. It's hard for me to define. I do disagree with Dr. Berg. There is a good example of X-linked dominant transmission in the XGA blood system as it is well known and easily testable. Now it's true there is Vitamin D resistant rickets which is another possibility of an X-link dominant gene, but not as well studied as the XGA system. If you find a specific kind of transmission, you have defined a genetically homogeneous disease. Because if the diseases are genetically heterogeneous they may be clinically heterogeneous too.

OTHER QUESTIONS FROM THE AUDIENCE

Spitzer: I shall first respond to some of the written questions directed to me from the audience.

Question: "When can we expect to receive DSM-III?"

Answer: The initial schedule was that it would be available January 1979 to coincide with the ICD 9. If the current plans are not changed because of controversy within the American Psychiatric Association, the plan is to have it available as a document for people who are doing field trials. And it will be generally available for anybody who wants to use it. But it will not be an official document until some time after January 1979 when it will be formally decided by the A.P.A. whether to make the DSM-III their official nomenclature.

Question: "Why are there so many omissions from the DSM-III section on organic mental disorders, i.e. specific syndrome such as neurosyphilis, epilepsy, cerebral tumor, etc?" The reason for this is that our system is consistent with the ICD 9. Whenever the aetiological agent is noted outside the mental disorders section, it has been noted mainly in neurology and would be coded on Axis 3. For example, neurosyphilis with dementia: the dementia would be noted as the psychiatric syndrome in Axis 3. Neurosyphilis would be noted as an infectious disorder in Axis 3.

Question: "Have there been any clinical neurologists serving as consultants in DSM-III?" The answer is yes, as of a week ago.

Question: "Why do we use the term cerebral vascular dementia?" This was something that was discussed at our DSM-III committee meeting. We define cerebral vascular dementia as a condition requiring focal neurological signs. Our difficulty is that there is always a somewhat artificial boundary between a neurological disorder and a psychiatric disorder. I don't think that this will be resolved very easily.

Question: "Can we really eliminate something like hysteria, and have we succumbed to pressure from the St. Louis group by having the term 'Briquet's disorder'?" No, actually we have not succumbed! We coined the term somatization disorder, which I think is a more acceptable term. The term "Briquet's disorder" is put in parentheses only to indicate that somatization refers to the condition that has been referred to as "Briquet's disorder." But the official term will be "somatization disorder."

Question: "Why don't we include in Axis 2 personality organization?"

I interpret this to mean: Why don't we include personality traits, i.e. non-disordered forms of personality functioning? We considered that possibility, but felt that it was too much of a task to have a nomenclature of non-disorders. So I think we will just suggest that, if it is useful, one should simply describe the personality traits, e.g., obsessional traits, which are short of a personality disorder.

Question: "Could you discuss Dr. Wender's concepts of borderline and how that will be elaborated into borderline personality disorder?" This is something that is still being worked on. I think, as I mentioned, we have identified six items which seem to correspond to the Wender, Kety, Rosenthal borderline schizophrenia. We have also added to that a list of 12 items which includes the more affective or Kernberg or Kohut type of borderline personality disorder. With those 18 items, we believe we can identify individuals whom people of a variety of persuasions will call borderline-something—probably, borderline personality disorder. Our next problem is, can we identify subtypes. There is one subtype which Wender would like us to call borderline schizophrenic personality. We are going to resist that suggestion very vigorously. I think we'd probably just end up by saying that there may be various subtypes of this borderline personality disorder, some of them having a genetic relationship to schizophrenia and some having a relationship to affective disorder. My own feeling is that I doubt they are that distinct. Dr. Wender said that his investigative group did not find these affective borderline items to be related genetically to schizophrenia. On the other hand, I think he will admit that his group was not really looking for them. When Dr. Jacobson did his interviews in Denmark, it seems clear that he was looking for mild schizophrenic symptomatology and he found it. I don't think it's really fair to say that he looked for the affective instability and lability—and did not find them. Now perhaps Dr. Wender will disagree, but that is my impression and I have read the cases, so I have some familiarity with them.

Question: "How do you relate the concept of symbiotic psychosis (Mahler's concept) to DSM-III?" The childhood disorders committee discussed that. They felt that infantile autism was a recognizable category. We have a category called early childhood psychosis which is probably closest to the symbiotic psychosis. There was one member of the childhood disorders committee who felt that we should have a separate category for Mahler's symbiotic psychosis. He was asked to provide us with clinical differentiating symptoms, but we have not heard from him.

Question: "Explain the difference between sub-acute and sub-chronic." We have defined the acute form of schizophrenia as an illness of less than three months, with total recovery. And we have defined the chronic variety as patients with continuing signs of the illness for at least two years. The sub-acute and the sub-chronic are just in-between categories.

Question: "What attempts have we made to correlate the underlying character disorder, i.e. conditions that would be noted on Axis 2, with the symptomatology for the acute schizophrenic episode?" The question refers to the attempts made to relate types of schizophrenic episodes to underlying personality patterns. Essentially, by having a multi-axial approach, it is possible with multiple diagnoses to denote those schizophrenics who started off with a schizoid personality and those who did not. Our approach is not to force this into a single diagnosis, but to express the same bits of information in a multi-axial diagnosis.

Grinker: I don't understand. Is the acute schizophrenic one whose duration of illness has been less than three months and has a total recovery? Now this must be a private world of yours. It does not conform to what actually happens to the acute schizophrenic. The episode may be deemed acute for a long time but he may never recover. He may continue into a chronic state. I appreciate the fact that you are taking the acute and the borderline schizophrenic out of DSM-III and I thank you very much for it. I also thank you very much for putting the borderline as a separate category. However, we then get into the acute because of the statement that the acute diagnosis is based on a duration of less than three months and has a total recovery. Well, that's just nonsense.

Spitzer: I do live in a private world, but I also live in a public world. The purpose of the three-month criterion for acute schizophrenia is to make it possible at any point of contact with a schizophrenic to characterize the couse up to that time. But only up to that time. So, obviously many patients who are given a diagnosis of acute schizophrenia, if this system is used, will eventually have been a sub-acute then a sub-chronic and eventually a chronic course. So I think there was a misunderstanding. The term acute at any moment in time means that either the patient has been ill for the first time for less than three months, and you don't know what's going to happen or the patient has had one or more previous episodes, none of which lasted more than three months, and from all of which he has recovered. Again it is an attempt to develop operational criteria.

Now, we are referring to the course of the illness treated or untreated. It's purely a descriptive statement. We have agonized over this because it is possible that one could have a total recovery that might have gone on to a chronic condition had there not been treatment. But since we can't eliminate treatment, and have no interest in doing so, we have to make our designations as they have occurred, whether or not there has been treatment. So it's purely a descriptive statement of the course at any moment in time.

van Praag: Very briefly, in reply to Dr. Grinker. I think the very reason that the term psychogenic psychosis or schizophreniform psychosis was used in Europe was that there are patients who develop acute psychotic symptoms with a strong schizophrenic color who had a very favorable prognosis. They do recover within weeks or months, and sometimes relapse, but not always. So I think that's the reason that in Europe the term schizophrenia is much more limited and terms like psychogenic psychosis are coined for what you call acute schizophrenia.

Winokur: I shall respond to a couple of questions from the floor which have not been dealt with in the previous questions.

Question: "We treat approximately 300 alcoholics (World Health Organization criteria) a year. Out of that number how many could we reasonably expect to have statistically determined affective disease? So far we seem to have found more well-defined schizophrenia in patients and families than affective illness. Would you recommend giving lithium to them all? And how much of the variance in the behavior of alcoholism does the genetics account for?" I can answer some of those questions very specifically. Regarding the percentage of alcoholics who have affective disorder out of 259 consecutively admitted alcoholics: 35 of them had an independently diagnosed affective disorder and 33 of them had an independently diagnosed antisocial personality. There was a scattering who had independently diagnosed schizophrenia, anxiety neurosis, organic brain syndromes of various sorts, etc. They were minimal and 159 out of them had primary alcoholism, i.e. they never had any evidence of a primary affective disorder which existed independently of the alcoholism.

Question: "Would you recommend giving lithium to acute schizophrenics?" All the studies that have been done, both blind and not blind, have shown an increased amount of remitting disorder in the families of acute schizophrenics. The only blind study that was ever done was done by myself and a group of associates and that one showed exactly the same thing. In fact it didn't even breed true. In that particular study, the schizo-affective or the acute schizophrenics had simple, ordinary affective disorder relatives diagnosed according to prespecified criteria. I think under these circumstances the relationship is clearly closer to affective disorder than it is to schizophrenia. I think it would be perfectly reasonable for a first attack to try to treat that person as if he or she had a remitting illness or an affective disorder. The fact is there are data to back it up anyway. Perris calls these people "cycloid psychosis" after Leonhard in Germany and he has very good data indicating the efficacy of lithium, both in treating and preventing subsequent episodes. And as I recall some of the patients in the NIMHA studies also showed efficacy for that.

Question: "How much of the variance in alcoholism is accounted for by genetic background?" I don't know the answer to that. I can tell you that in any good study in which there may be three or four families of alcoholic probands, you find that alcoholic probands have about 25 to 30 percent of their male relatives affected with the same disease, but there are always a certain number of alcoholics who have no alcoholism in their family. As I recall, Goodwin and Guze did a very small study in St. Louis which indicated that if you took a group of alcoholics they were more likely to have teetotallers in their family than a group of non-alcoholics. So that is the kind of problem you have. Obviously, the cause of alcoholism is alcohol and if they don't drink you can't make the diagnosis and there will be some people who for some reason or another don't drink. Now that's unfortunately a noise in the system. I don't know how you get by with it. The fact is that if you look at a group of alcoholics you will find a very high proportion who have alcoholic first-degree relatives. And there are two adoption studies now. One was done in the north of Sweden by Bowman, the other was the Guze, Goodwin, Hermansen, Schulsinger, Winokur study. The latter was a blind adoption study which showed a quite significant increase in alcoholism in the adopted children of alcoholic parents over controls.

My confidence in asserting that there is a genetic factor in alcoholism is based on having done a study in which we subjected 259 consecutively admitted alcoholics to a systematic interview and made diagnosis on the basis of the results of the systematic interview according to prestated criteria. I think that genetic studies are of interest to psychiatrists only to help in diagnosis and I think that we will separate out specific kinds of illnesses by the use of genetic studies rather than getting specific illnesses and doing genetic studies on them. It is another methodology, but it is as valid as the clinical picture, the course of the illness, or the response to treatment.

Feinstein: What troubles me, Dr. Winokur, is that about a century and a half ago, Prof. Bruset of Paris could have said with enormous confidence: "I have done blood letting in 327 people with sore throats and of those 327, 292 recovered beautifully. Therefore, blood letting is superb treatment." And he could say just as well, "I have observed, I have counted, I have reported, and therefore I am right." The mere act of counting and observation does not necessarily assure that what you are observing and counting is correct.

Spitzer: Well, I don't think the historical analogy that you gave, which involves a methodological flaw which we are well aware of, namely a lack of experimental design sufficient to make a causal inference, really is the same problem that Dr. Winokur may or may not have. So I would have to come to the defense of Dr. Winokur there.

NEUROBIOLOGICAL QUESTIONS

van Praag: Question: "Have studies been done looking for familial patterns of depressive illness in relatives of patients with low and normal serotonin turnover?" *Question:* "Is there any correlation between the low 5-hydroxyindoleacetic acid depressives and the depressive sub-group with low level of metabolites of norepinephrine such as MHPG in their CSF?"

Well the first question of course is a most fascinating topic. Suppose it would be true that low 5-hydroxyindoleacetic acid is a kind of a vulnerability factor. I would be interested in studying the families of these patients, but of course it is not an easy task to convince the family of a patient suffering from recurring depression to be admitted into hospital for a lumbar puncture. I am not aware so far of any study accomplishing this, although I think it a very important and very intriguing question. Regarding the second question I think you will have to differentiate first between CSF MHPG and urinary MHPG. Unfortunately, the correlation between the two is very low. It is very difficult to explain. Maybe one of the reasons is that MHPG and lumbar CSF is mainly derived from the spinal cord and not from higher levels. But the correlation with depression has been found mostly with urinary MHPG and not much with CSF MHPG. Regarding the relationship between serotonin and noradrenalin in depression, it's more likely that disturbances of 5-HT (Serotonin) and noradrenalin are separate; that you really have the 5-HT subgroup and noradrenalin subgroup. However, I think the number of patients studied so far is too small to make any definite statement about this particular question.

Reitan: Question: "How helpful are your organicity tests with children; if they are helpful what would be the indication for administering these tests to children?" I started on development of measures for evaluation of brain behavior relationships in children in 1951. At that time there were very little data. There were very few procedures available and, in fact, we have worked very intensivly in developing methods for children. Our methods with children, I think, are less well known and certainly less widely used than our methods with adult subjects. We have three batteries of tests: one for children age 5 through 8; another for children 9 through 14; and the adult tests which can be administered generally to persons 15 and older. We find that we are just about on the verge of being able to formulate, in explicit terms, a neuropsychological diagnosis of learning disabilities supported by specific, objectively obtained measurements. We also find that we can, in many instances, use our data as a basis for evaluating the cognitive structure of the child as it relates to his predisposition to display various types of behavioral difficulties. We have developed a method for obtaining descriptive data that has been tested and validated by its degree of relationship or predictive significance particularly to the point that Dr. Feinstein mentioned. We make these predictions in each of these directions with respect to aetiology and pathogenesis. In relation to other symptoms or classifications and with respect to prognosis, I believe that our measurements in children have significance in each of these directions that goes well beyond chance.

DIAGNOSTIC CLASSIFICATIONS

Question: "Is there any collaboration going on between IPSS and the development of DSM-III?"

Spitzer: The IPSS is the International Pilot Study of Schizophrenia which is a W.H.O. sponsored study of schizophrenia. Perhaps the question is about the relationship to ICD 9. Perhaps I didn't make that clear. The mental disorders section or chapter of the International Classification of Diseases 9 has already been completed. It is such a large effort involving committees from different countries that they have to have the draft document ready several years before it is used. So they have had a draft version which I believe has gone through all the revisions. It has been available to our committee for the last year or two. So essentially we have had input from them and we have looked at their categories and have made changes in the classification only when we thought there were good reasons for doing it. We have also received comments from individuals who have participated in that group—for example, John Wing as well as Michael Rutter, who is an expert in the area of childhood diagnosis. Our initial feeling was that we were somewhat anxious that our ICD colleagues would take a jaundiced view of our tinkering with the ICD 9, but we've had the feeling that they respect our efforts and feel that what we are doing in making revision in ICD 9 may be useful in the development of ICD 10.

The specific research findings coming out of the IPSS study have certainly very decisively influenced our definition of schizophrenia. We relied very extensively on the findings concerning the central core concept of schizophrenia which we have built into our definition and we have relied on the supporting research data to justify the use of that definition. It is a more restrictive concept of schizophrenia than many American psychiatrists have been comfortable with. However, I think over the years after the US/UK study and the IPSS study most American psychiatrists are prepared to accept the more restrictive definition only if it will be useful in helping communication and providing a basis for research studies which up to now have been very difficult to accomplish.

Feinstein: I wonder, Dr. Spitzer, why you have tied yourself to something as intellectually decadent as unverified, unvalidated and untested as the ICD criteria. The only thing that it has to sustain it is the sheer weight of inertia, tradition and the regular meetings of the group of people who juggle names around without ever checking out how they get used. What kind of transference can someone work out for your group that will liberate you from those shackles.

Spitzer: What would you have done if you were chairman of the ICD 9 committee? Part of the reason we have shackled our star to a broken-down chariot is that there is a treaty obligation the United States government has with the World Health Organization to collect morality and morbidity statistics using the international classification of diseases. When we started on DSM-III a little more than two years ago, we perceived that the mandate was to develop the best classification possible, and only secondarily to worry about our compatibility because of this treaty obligation. Our initial feeling was that this was going to make it very difficult for us to be creative. Through the procedure of allowing ourselves two extra digits, we found that we could really do just about anything we wanted to and still be compatible. Now you ask why we accept the ICD criteria. We haven't really found that using ICD 9 as a starting point has cramped our style. Dr. Feinstein, I would ask you this question since I've got the floor. What would you do if you had the task of revising or providing some kind of international classification? I assume that one of the things you would do is what we've been doing, which is developing criteria, but would you abandon the notion of categories of illness or what?

Feinstein: Well, I think the first step would be to try to establish operational criteria for the terms. As it currently stands, those terms are like a bunch of labels in a grocery store that has been flooded and all the cans have had the labels washed off; you agree on what the labels are but you have no idea what's in the cans. That's the fundamental fault of the ICD. Secondly they shuffle labels around in various arbitrary ways. This is bizarre. In 1920 a person who had cardiac and renal disease would be quoted as having cardiac disease. In 1930 they reshuffle it and that person is then quoted as having renal disease. It's a kind of hierarchical anarchy that the ICD is engaged in. There has been no careful clinical attention to what are the contents of any of these things. If the ICD is simply a kind of international stock market which juggles the names of stocks around, that's fine. But if you want to regard that as a scientific qualification, you have to begin with verified aspects of what goes into it and not just alter the labels.

Wing: I just want to say that Dr. Feinstein has probably been talking about the ICD as a whole and not the psychiatric section of it which is Section 5. In fact, there is a glossary of definitions so it's not a question of just a grab bag. There is a definition of the various concepts used; in fact, that glossary has itself been revised. It's now in the second edition and with the tenth revision I hope there will be an even better one—which will be better because of DSM-III. It is improving all the time and what one mustn't lose sight of in this kind of work is that the basic idea of having this kind of international classification is to increase communicability between physicians. You will never get that if you try to impose one set of criteria from one country even though it may very well be the best set possible at the time. It simply can't be done. It has to be done by a process of negotiation and your suggestion that you should bring in politicians to do this is not such a bad notion. It is in fact a matter of politics to some extent. If certain countries say that they want this particular syndrome included, then you can't offend them. Otherwise you won't get them to use the classification. And I think it is useful to use the classification even with all its imperfections. What I would like to end this comment with is the feeling that there is some progress in this field. We are in fact getting better at it and I think DSM-III is part of that process of improvement.

Index